Choose this not that

for

High Triglycerides

by

Personal Remedies

Published by Simple Software Publishing.

Copyright © 2016 by Personal Remedies, LLC
5 Oregon Street
Georgetown, MA 01833 USA

Second Edition

ISBN-13: 978-0-9652457-3-9   ISBN-10: 0-9652457-3-X

Printed by CreateSpace.

Choose this not that

for

High Triglycerides

Inside this book, you will find a list of food items and easy to follow suggestions on how to improve your health through nutrition and the food choices you make every day.

Suggestions are provided for those with high triglycerides or those who are prone to develop this condition.

In addition, the book contains similar information for those who have one of the following common health conditions or risks along with high triglycerides:

- Alzheimer's disease
- Cancer risk
- Depression
- Diabetes (Type 2)
- Excess body weight or Obesity
- Gout
- Heart Disease
- High blood pressure
- High cholesterol
- Stress
- Vitamin D deficiency

Table of Contents

Important Notes

The purpose of this book is to provide helpful and informative material and to educate. It is in no way intended as substitute for medical advice. We recommend in all cases that you contact your personal doctor or health care provider before you embark upon any new diet or treatment of yourself.

This book is sold with the understanding that the publisher, the author and the distributor of this book are neither liable, nor have responsibility to any person or entity with respect to any loss, damage or injury which is incurred as a consequence, directly or indirectly, of the use or application of any of the contents of this book.

How to use this book

The guidelines presented on the following pages are for an adult male or female. They do not apply to children, pregnant women or breast feeding mothers.

Our suggestions are organized by food groups. Within each food group, **items are presented in a specific and deliberate order**. In the case of recommended items (those that could <u>improve</u> your health), the most helpful remedies or suggestions are presented first. In the case of items to avoid (those that could <u>worsen</u> your conditions), the most critical ones to avoid are listed first. The items that are suggested under <u>Instead Choose</u>, are likely to be neutral for your health (i.e., neither improve nor worsen your conditions) based on the information available to us at the time.

Unfortunately, health issues often come our way in groups of two or more. If we are obese or under stress, then chances are we are also at risk with a number of other health issues such as cancer, high blood pressure, or Vitamin D deficiency. If we have Vitamin D deficiency then chances are we either suffer from or have higher risk of getting Osteoporosis, Crohn's disease or kidney problems. Each health issue often results in other health complications, thus the need for looking at a combination of health concerns and risks when formulating our nutrition plans and lifestyle changes. It is for that reason, that we have included separate guidelines for those who might suffer from the most likely and common combinations of health issues related to the main health concern addressed by this book.

One of the factors that make *Choose This not That* series of publications different from all others available to you in the market is that we offer nutrition guidelines for likely COMBINATIONS of illnesses and risks that may be relevant to your situation. We also give you specific guidance by telling you exactly which fish, fruit, vegetable, nut ... is the best for you as well as listing the worst items. We give you an ordered list of food items within each food group, not just a food group.

We have listed alternative therapies and herbal medicines relevant (either helpful or harmful) to your condition. But it is beyond the scope of this book to provide specific guidelines on dosage or how to best benefit from these options. We encourage you to explore these alternatives with your natural health care provider.

Our approach in the *Choose This not That* series is to help people improve or combat their health issues through nutrition (i.e., consumption of food items that they can easily find in their local grocery store), exercise and lifestyle changes. We accomplish that through identification of those items that can improve your health, those that can worsen it, and those that play a neutral role. We trust that you can use this information to alter your diet and lifestyle choices to improve your health and wellbeing.

Serving Sizes

Except for what is noted below, our standard serving size for most foods is 100 grams or 3.5 ounces. For most liquids, it is about half a cup.

For nuts and seeds, the standard serving size is 30 grams (approximately an ounce). For dried fruits, the standard serving size is 25 grams.

For butter, margarine, various oils & fats, fresh herbs (e.g., basil, parsley), crackers, uncooked grains or flour, fresh hot peppers, condiments (e.g., ketchup, mustard, pickles), sugar and salad dressings ... the standard serving size is 20 grams (which in many cases corresponds to one table spoon).

For dry herbs, spices, salt, pepper and the like, the standard serving size is 2 grams (which in most cases corresponds to less than one tea spoon).

Please follow preparation guidelines for herbal supplements, and use a serving size appropriate for the specific use of the herb. Please use caution when selecting these supplements since they are not subject to FDA regulations.

Fruits and vegetables are normally assumed to be served raw. Various fish, seafood and meats are normally assumed to be cooked.

How we developed the content of this book

To provide specific and actionable information and guidance on food choices that you make every day and how they might impact your health, we had to quantify a relative level of goodness (or badness) for every individual food item in our database as they relate to each specific illness or health concern tracked in our system.

Most food and nutrition related research and publications in the U.S. are focused on vitamins, minerals, micro-nutrients, and substances such as cholesterol, fat and fiber. And to a lesser extent there are studies and data on herbal remedies, alternative and complementary medicine, and non-western treatments.

There is not enough data or widely accepted studies that focus on individual foods (e.g., watermelon, white fish and walnuts) and how they relate to specific illnesses or health risks. Our goal has been to help address that void.

Here is a very brief description of our approach:

a) We maintain detailed nutrition information on every individual food item in our system. Most of such data is available from the U.S. Department of Agriculture. And for some data (e.g., Mercury, Gluten) we have found other reliable sources.

b) When there is data available on health benefits (or adverse impact) of a specific food item, or nutrient (e.g., vitamins, minerals) we capture and make use of such data.

c) If a given nutrient is good for a health condition (e.g., Vitamin A is good for night blindness), then all food items that are rich in that nutrient (Vitamin A) are given a positive/higher rating as they relate to that condition (night blindness). Similarly if a given nutrient has adverse impact on a health condition then all food items that contain that nutrient are given a negative/lower rating.

d) Some food items contain much more of a nutrient than others. Our technology takes that into account.

e) Some nutrients are found to be much more effective (e.g., Vitamin A) than some other nutrient (e.g., Zinc) as they relate to a given health condition (e.g., night blindness). Our technology distinguishes between the two.

f) Sometimes a study or a source behind the relationship between a nutrient and a health condition is much more reliable than another. Our approach is sensitive to that.

g) Certain nutrients facilitate absorption of another nutrient (e.g., Vitamin D facilitates absorption of Calcium). We make use of such information. For example, let's say Calcium is good for Tooth Development. Then all food items that are rich in Vitamin D are given a more positive consideration as they relate to Tooth Development.

h) Similarly some substances may reduce absorption of or increase the need for another (e.g., Caffeine may increase the need for Calcium). In the above example, all food items that contain Caffeine will receive a negative/lower rating as they relate to Tooth Development.

i) Our process and the steps mentioned above are automated by our unique (proprietary) and patented technology. At the conclusion of our process, there is a single score that represents the level of goodness or badness for every food item as it relates to each health condition maintained in our system. These scores are the basis for all the sorted lists of food items that you find in the Choose This not That series of publications.

j) For multiple conditions, the sum of these scores is what drives the ranking of the food items and our guidelines.

In closing, it is important to note that in these publications we are not making scientific claims, nor do we suggest perfection of our approach. Our goal is to simply provide a significant improvement over status-quo. No human being or health care specialist can properly and fully take into account the enormity, complexity and contradictions inherent in the interrelationships of food, health, genetics, environment, exercise, lifestyle, etc. that affect our wellbeing. We have merely attempted to use the power of technology to provide you much better and more relevant information to maintain healthier living.

High Triglycerides (HT)

Triglycerides are a type of fat that exist in the bloodstream, in fat tissues and in foods. Triglycerides can be produced from fats in the foods we consume, from carbohydrates, or from calories not used by the tissues immediately after consumption and stored in the fat cells for future use.

High level of triglycerides in the blood can result in hardening and narrowing of arteries, leading to greater possibility of heart attack and strokes. This condition often occurs along with high level of cholesterol in the blood stream. It is often discovered in the same blood test that measures cholesterol level. Triglycerides level is considered high if it is greater than 200 milligrams per deci-liter.

The most likely causes for having high triglycerides are:
- drinking too much alcohol,
- being overweight,
- consuming too much sugars and carbohydrates
- suffering from other medical conditions such as diabetes or kidney failure

Proper nutrition and exercise can be very effective in lowering the triglycerides level in your blood.

Choose these for High Triglycerides

Top 5 items to choose:

Fish Oil; Wild Fish; Shellfish; Garlic & Ginger; Soybeans; & Exercise;

Food items and actions that could improve your health (within a food group, most helpful items are listed first):

Meat, Fish & Poultry

Anchovy; **Bluefish**; **Cisco (smoked)**; **Mackerel**; **Mackerel (king)**; **Marlin**; **Salmon (pink)**; **Spot**; **Sturgeon**; **Swordfish**; **Trout**; **Tuna (blue fin)**; **White fish**; **Herring**; **Sablefish**; **Tilefish**; **Caviar**; **Salmon (smoked, Lox)**; **Mussels**; **Bass (striped)**; **Smelt**; **Tuna (yellowfin)**; **Halibut**; **Bass (seabass)**; **Wolffish**; **Pollock**; **Sucker**; **Mullet**; **Bass (freshwater)**; **Drum**; **Oysters**; **Whiting**; **Lobster (spiny)**; **Shad**; **Crab (Dungeness)**; **Milkfish**; **Yellowtail**; **Cisco**; **Crab (Alaskan King)**; **Surimi**; **Pompano fish**; **Crab (snow)**; Tilapia; Clams; Dolphinfish (Mahi-Mahi); Seatrout; Walleye; Octopus; White fish (smoked); Grouper; Snapper; Flatfish (flounder & sole); Butterfish; Scup; Catfish; Fish roe; Lingcod; Chicken breast (no skin); Lobster; Burbot; Rockfish; Cusk; Carp; Perch; Haddock; Northern pike; Cod; Veal loin; Scallops; Pheasant breast; Ling; Monkfish; Sheepshead; Crab (Blue); Veal shank; Quail breast; Pumpkinseed sunfish; Turbot; Conch; Orange roughy; Pout; Snail; Cuttlefish; Shrimp; Tuna (canned); Beef filet mignon; Caribou meat; Crayfish;

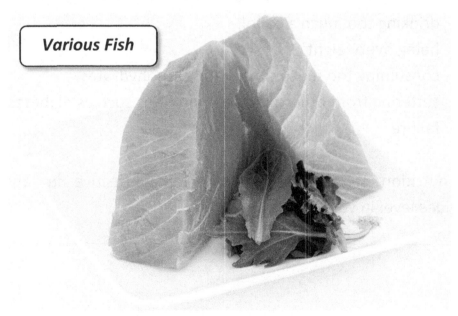

Various Fish

Eggs, Beans, Nuts and Seeds

Soybeans (dried); Seeds (chia); Egg substitute; Seeds (flaxseed);

Fruits & Juices

In general, there are no fruits or juices that can <u>lower</u> your Triglycerides. But there are certain fruits or juices that may be neutral for your High Triglycerides condition, which are listed in the next section.

Vegetables

Garlic; Various Mushrooms; Artichoke; Onions; Winged beans leaves; Peppers (jalapeno); Peppers (pimento); Arrowroot; Chicory greens; Taro leaves; Fiddlehead ferns; Tomatoes (sun-dried); Peppers;

Breads, Grains, Cereals, Pasta

Rice bran; Rice cakes (Brown rice); Wheat bran; Oats; Triticale;

Dairy Products, Fats & Oils

Fish oil (cod liver); **Other Fish oil**; Oil (olive); Oil (flaxseed);

Desserts, Snacks, Beverages

Tea (green); Red Bull (drink);

Herbs & Spices, Fast Foods, Prepared Foods

Ginger; Cayenne (red) pepper; Cinnamon; Fish stock; Soup (clam chowder); Miso; Kimchi;

Alternative Therapies & Miscellaneous

Wild fish and free range animals; **Exercise of various forms including cardiovascular and weight training;**

Key Nutrients & Herbal Meds

Omega-3 fatty acids; **Vitamin B-3 (Niacin; in nicotinic acid form; not recommended as supplement or drug)**; Guggul; Vitamin B-5 (Pantothenic Acid; in pantethine form);

Do not choose these for High Triglycerides

Top 5 items to avoid:

Whole Milk; Egg Yolk; Fast Foods; Sweets; Butter, Margarine & Hydrogenated vegetable oil;

Avoid or consume much less of the following (within a food group, most harmful items are listed first):

Meat, Fish & Poultry

Bacon; Beef (cured brkfst strips); Beef jerky sticks; Organ Meats; Salami; Bologna; Chicken skin; Chorizo; Frankfurters; Luncheon meats; Pepperoni; Pork breakfast strips; Pork headcheese; Pork ribs; Pork skins; Pork spare ribs; Sausages; Turkey skins; Goose; Pastrami; Lamb ribs; Beef chuck/brisket; Pork; Chicken wings; Beef (ground); Beef ribs; Chicken dark meat; Corned beef; Lamb; Beaver meat; Beef; Squab (pigeon); Bear meat; Quail; Croaker; Bison/buffalo meat; Frog legs; Boar meat; Duck (no skin); Goat meat; Rabbit meat; Pheasant; Abalone;

Instead choose: **Squid (Calamari); Turkey breast; Sardines; Veal shoulder; Shark; Venison; Eel; Turkey dark meat; Whelk; Guinea hen;**

Eggs, Beans, Nuts and Seeds

Egg yolk; Brazil nuts; Butternuts; Hickory nuts; Pili nuts; Pine nuts; Seeds: cottonseed, pumpkin/squash, sesame, watermelon, safflower; Almonds; Beechnuts; Pecans; Pistachio nuts; Cashew nuts; Walnuts (black); Seeds (sunflower); Egg (hard-boiled); Peanuts; Walnuts; Egg (raw); Hazelnuts or Filberts; Coconut meat (dried); Coconut meat (raw); Acorns; Egg (duck); Chickpeas; Beans (winged); Coconut milk; Beans (baked); Cornnuts; Soybeans (green); Lupin; Chestnuts; Soy milk; Macadamia nuts; Other Beans; Black-eyed peas; Pigeon peas;

Instead choose: **Alfalfa sprouts; Peas (sugar/snap); Peas (green); Ginkgo nuts; Egg white; Lentils; Peas (split); Seeds (breadnut tree); Breadfruit seeds;**

Fruits & Juices

Tamarind; Avocado; Longans; Plantains; Currants (dried); Dates; Figs; Grapes; Litchi; Dried Fruits; Prune juice; Banana; Breadfruit; Cherries; Pomegranate; Quince; Raisins; Rowal; Abiyuch; Kumquats; Pears; Apples; Cranberry juice; Grape juice; Mango; Persimmons; Pomegranate juice; Tangerines; Passion fruit; Apple juice; Apricots; Blueberries; Boysenberries; Cantaloupe; Currants (raw); Durian; Elderberries; Grapefruit; Grapefruit juice; Guava; Honeydew melon; Jujube (fruit); Kiwi fruit; Loganberry; Mulberries; Nectarine; Oranges; Papaya; Peaches; Pineapple; Pineapple juice; Plum; Watermelon;

Instead choose: **Acerola; Blackberries; Cowberries; Cranberries; Gooseberries; Lemon; Lime; Natal Plum (Carissa); Olives; Orange juice; Pitanga; Pumelo (Shaddock); Raspberries; Rhubarb; Starfruit; Strawberries;**

Vegetables

Peppers (ancho); Artichoke (Jerusalem); Shallots; Sweet potatoes; Arrowhead; Beets; Lotus root; Potatoes w/skin; Taro; Yam;

*Instead **choose**: Broccoli; Cauliflower; Endive; Kelp; Squash (Acorn); other vegetables;*

Breads, Grains, Cereals, Pasta

Cereal (wheat germ); Biscuits; Bread (banana); Bread (cornbread); Cereal (granola); Croissant; Danish pastry; Donuts; Granola bars; Muffins (blueberry); Muffins (oat bran); Muffins (wheat bran); Sweet rolls; Waffles; Muffins (corn); Crackers (wheat); Rolls (whole-wheat dinner); Bread sticks; Noodles (Chinese chow Mein); Crackers (milk); Crackers (whole-wheat); Cereal (bran flakes); Rolls (Kaiser); Cereal (raisin bran); Melba toast; Tortillas (corn); Wheat germ; Cereal (shredded wheat); Crackers (saltines); Rolls (hamburger/hot dog); Various Bread; Bagels; English muffins; Noodles (egg); Various cereals; Amaranth; Quinoa; Rolls (French); Spelt; Bulgur; Millet; Rice (brown); Rice (wild); Spaghetti (whole-wheat); Toasted bread; English muffins (whole-wheat); Barley; Pasta; Spaghetti; Corn; Corn bran; Couscous; Crackers (matzo); Noodles (Japanese); Noodles (rice); Rye grain; Wheat;

*Instead **choose**: Rice (white); Spaghetti (spinach);Buckwheat; Croutons; Durum wheat; Oat bran; Semolina; Sorghum grain; Whole-wheat; Bread (wheat germ); Bread (French/Sourdough);*

Dairy Products, Fats & Oils

Milk (whole); Butter; Various Cheese; Cheese spread; Cream (whipped); Fat (chicken, duck, turkey); Hydrogenated vegetable oil; Lard; Margarine; Margarine-like spreads; Non-dairy creamers; Various Oils; Vegetable shortening; Milk (chocolate); Fat (beef/lamb/pork); Sour cream; Milk (skim); Milk (1% fat); Milk (2% fat); Buttermilk; Whey (sweet); Cheese (Cottage); Cream; Yogurt;

Desserts, Snacks, Beverages

Sherbet; After-dinner mints; Brownies; Cakes; Candies; Cheesecake; Chewing gum; Chocolate mousse; Coffee liqueur; Coffeecake; Cookies; Cream puffs/Éclair; Crème de menthe; Dessert toppings; Frostings; Fruit leather/rolls; Halvah (candy); Honey; Ice creams; Ice cream cones; Jams & Preserves; Jellies; Marshmallows; Peanut butter; Pies; Pie crust; Popcorn (oil popped); Potato sticks; Puff pastry; Taro chips; Tortilla chips; Potato chips; Frozen yogurt; Molasses; Popcorn (air popped); Pudding; Chocolate (sweet); Piña colada; Milk shakes; Chocolate (dark); Pancakes; Eggnog; Applesauce; Soft (carbonated) drinks; Ginger ale; Hot chocolate; Tonic water; Pretzels; 80+ proof distilled alc. bev.; Fruit punch; Lemonade; Whiskey; Sports drinks; Wine (red); Wine (white); Malted drinks (nonalcoholic); Beer;

*Instead **choose**: Coffee; Coffee (decaf); Orange juice; Tea (herbal); Tea (plain); Tomato juice; Water;*

Herbs & Spices, Fast Foods, Prepared Foods

Breaded shrimp; Cheeseburger; Foie gras or liver pate; French toast; Hash brown potatoes; Hush puppies; Nachos; Onion rings; Pizza; Potato pancakes; Potato salad; Salad dressings; Syrup (chocolate); **Taco shells; Tahini; Syrup (maple); Hot dog; French fries; Syrup (sorghum); Natto; Hamburger; Syrup (table blends); Egg rolls (veg); Hummus; Sausage (meatless); Teriyaki sauce; Mayonnaise; Cottonseed meal; Tofu (fried); Sugar (brown); Sugar (table, powder); Chicken Nuggets; Soy sauce**; Cornmeal (whole-grain); Syrup (malt); Corn cakes; Barbecue sauce; Tofu; Falafel; Sugar (maple); Pickle (sweet); Poppy seed; Sauce (Hoisin); Tempeh; Beef broth & stock; Chicken broth & stock; Soup (beef barley); Soup (chicken noodle); Soup (veg/beef); Cole slaw; Ketchup; Macaroni;

Instead* choose: *Balsamic vinegar; Herbs & Spices; Horseradish; Mustard; Pickle; Salt & Pepper; Sauces; Sauerkraut; Tomato paste; Vinegar; Succotash;

Alternative Therapies & Miscellaneous

Cheese made w/whole milk; Deep-fried foods; Excess body weight; Corn syrup; Smoking/Tobacco; 2+ alcoholic drinks/day; Artificial sweeteners; Baking using butter;

Key Nutrients & Herbal Meds

Trans fatty acids; Omega-6 fatty acid (LA); Fat (saturated); Alcohol; Carbohydrates; Cholesterol; Sugar (refined); Sugar (total);

Look-up Table – Food Suitability for HT

Food Item or Other	Suitability for HT	Remarks (if any)
1-2 alcoholic drinks/day	Consume less	
2+ alcoholic drinks/day	Consume less	
80+ proof distilled alc. bev.	Consume less	
Abalone	Consume less	
Abiyuch	Consume less	
Acerola	Neutral/OK	
Acorns	Consume much less	
After-dinner mints	Avoid	
Alcohol	Consume less	
Alfalfa sprouts	Neutral/OK	
Almonds	Avoid	
Amaranth	Consume less	
Amaranth leaves	Neutral/OK	
Anchovy	Most helpful	
Apple juice	Consume less	
Apples	Consume less	
Apples (dried)	Consume less	
Applesauce	Consume much less	
Apricots	Consume less	
Apricots (dried)	Consume less	
Arrowhead	Consume less	
Arrowroot	Helpful	
Artichoke	Helpful	
Artichoke (Jerusalem)	Consume less	
Artificial sweeteners	Consume less	
Arugula	Neutral/OK	
Asparagus	Neutral/OK	
Aspartame (Equal)	Consume less	
Avocado	Consume much less	
Bacon	Avoid	
Bagels	Consume less	
Baking using butter	Consume less	
Balsam pear	Neutral/OK	
Balsam pear leafy tips	Neutral/OK	
Balsamic vinegar	Neutral/OK	
Banana	Consume less	
Banana (dried)	Consume less	
Barbecue sauce	Consume less	
Barley	Consume less	
Basil (fresh)	Neutral/OK	
Bass (freshwater)	More helpful	
Bass (seabass)	Most helpful	
Bass (striped)	Most helpful	
Beans (adzuki)	Consume less	
Beans (baked)	Consume less	
Beans (black)	Consume less	
Beans (fava)	Consume less	
Beans (Great Northern)	Consume less	

Food Item or Other	Suitability for HT	Remarks (if any)
Beans (hyacinth)	Consume less	
Beans (kidney)	Consume less	
Beans (lima)	Neutral/OK	
Beans (moth beans)	Consume less	
Beans (mung)	Consume less	
Beans (navy)	Consume less	
Beans (pinto)	Consume less	
Beans (winged)	Consume less	
Beans (yardlong)	Neutral/OK	
Beans (yellow)	Consume less	
Bear meat	Consume much less	
Beaver meat	Consume much less	
Beechnuts	Avoid	
Beef (cured brkfst strips)	Avoid	
Beef (cured dried)	Consume much less	
Beef (ground)	Avoid	
Beef brain	Consume much less	
Beef broth	Consume less	
Beef chuck/brisket	Avoid	
Beef filet mignon	Helpful	
Beef heart	Avoid	
Beef jerky sticks	Avoid	
Beef kidneys	Avoid	
Beef liver	Consume much less	
Beef rib eye	Consume less	
Beef ribs	Consume much less	
Beef round steak	Consume less	
Beef shank	Consume much less	
Beef spleen	Avoid	
Beef stock	Consume less	
Beef tenderloin/Tbone/portrhse	Consume less	
Beef tongue	Avoid	
Beef top sirloin	Consume less	
Beer	Consume less	
Beerwurst beer salami	Avoid	
Beet greens	Neutral/OK	
Beets	Consume less	
Bell peppers (green)	Neutral/OK	
Bell peppers (red)	Neutral/OK	
Birth control pills	Neutral/OK	
Biscuits	Avoid	
Bison/buffalo meat	Consume less	
Blackberries	Neutral/OK	
Black-eyed peas	Consume less	
Blueberries	Consume less	
Bluefish	Most helpful	
Boar meat	Consume less	
Bok choy	Neutral/OK	
Bologna (various)	Avoid	
Borage	Neutral/OK	

Food Item or Other	Suitability for HT	Remarks (If any)
Boysenberries	Consume less	
Brazil nuts	Avoid	
Bread (banana)	Avoid	
Bread (cornbread)	Avoid	
Bread (French/Sourdough)	Neutral/OK	
Bread (Italian)	Consume less	
Bread (oat bran)	Consume less	
Bread (pumpernickel)	Consume less	
Bread (wheat germ)	Neutral/OK	
Bread (white)	Consume less	
Bread (whole-wheat)	Consume less	
Bread sticks	Avoid	
Breaded shrimp	Avoid	
Breadfruit	Consume less	
Breadfruit seeds	Neutral/OK	
Broccoli	Neutral/OK	
Broccoli (Chinese)	Neutral/OK	
Brownies	Avoid	
Brussels sprouts	Neutral/OK	
Buckwheat	Neutral/OK	
Bulgur	Consume less	
Burbot	Helpful	
Butter (salted)	Avoid	
Butter (unsalted)	Avoid	
Butterfish	Helpful	
Buttermilk	Consume less	
Butternuts	Avoid	
Cabbage (green)	Neutral/OK	
Cabbage (red)	Neutral/OK	
Cabbage (savoy)	Neutral/OK	
Cake (angel food)	Avoid	
Cake (Boston cream pie)	Avoid	
Cake (chocolate)	Avoid	
Cake (gingerbread)	Avoid	
Cake (pound)	Avoid	
Cake (shortcake)	Avoid	
Cake (sponge)	Avoid	
Cake (yellow)	Avoid	
Candies (caramel)	Avoid	
Candies (hard)	Avoid	
Candies (peanut bar)	Avoid	
Candies (peanut brittle)	Avoid	
Candies (sesame crunch)	Avoid	
Canned foods	Consume less	
Cantaloupe	Consume less	
Capers	Neutral/OK	
Carbohydrates	Consume less	
Cardamom	Neutral/OK	
Caribou meat	Helpful	
Carob (candy)	Avoid	

Food Item or Other	Suitability for HT	Remarks (if any)
Carp	Helpful	
Carrots	Neutral/OK	
Cashew nuts	Avoid	
Catfish	Helpful	
Cauliflower	Neutral/OK	
Caviar	Most helpful	
Cayenne (red) pepper	Helpful	
Celery	Neutral/OK	
Celtuce	Neutral/OK	
Cereal (bran flakes)	Consume much less	
Cereal (corn flakes)	Consume less	
Cereal (cream of wheat)	Consume less	
Cereal (granola)	Avoid	
Cereal (raisin bran)	Consume much less	
Cereal (rice crisps)	Consume less	
Cereal (shredded wheat)	Consume less	
Cereal (wheat germ)	Avoid	
Cereal (whole-wheat)	Consume less	
Cheese (American)	Avoid	
Cheese (Blue)	Avoid	
Cheese (Brie)	Avoid	
Cheese (Camembert)	Avoid	
Cheese (Cheddar)	Avoid	
Cheese (Colby)	Avoid	
Cheese (Cottage)	Consume less	
Cheese (Cream)	Avoid	
Cheese (Edam)	Avoid	
Cheese (Feta)	Avoid	
Cheese (Fontina)	Avoid	
Cheese (Gjetost)	Avoid	
Cheese (Goat)	Avoid	
Cheese (Gouda)	Avoid	
Cheese (Gruyere)	Avoid	
Cheese (Limburger)	Avoid	
Cheese (Mozzarella)	Avoid	
Cheese (Parmesan)	Avoid	
Cheese (Pimento)	Avoid	
Cheese (Port de salut)	Avoid	
Cheese (Ricotta)	Consume much less	
Cheese (Romano)	Avoid	
Cheese (Roquefort)	Avoid	
Cheese (Swiss)	Avoid	
Cheese made w/whole milk	Avoid	
Cheese spread	Avoid	
Cheeseburger	Avoid	
Cheesecake	Avoid	
Cherries	Consume less	
Chervil	Neutral/OK	
Chestnuts	Consume less	
Chewing gum	Avoid	

Food Item or Other	Suitability for HT	Remarks (if any)
Chicken breast (no skin)	Helpful	
Chicken broth	Consume less	
Chicken dark meat	Consume much less	
Chicken giblets	Consume much less	
Chicken heart	Avoid	
Chicken liver	Consume much less	
Chicken Nuggets	Consume much less	
Chicken skin	Avoid	
Chicken stock	Consume less	
Chicken wings	Avoid	
Chickpeas	Consume much less	
Chicory greens	Helpful	
Chives	Neutral/OK	
Chocolate (dark)	Consume much less	
Chocolate (sweet)	Avoid	
Chocolate mousse	Avoid	
Cholesterol	Consume less	
Chorizo	Avoid	
Chrysanthemum (Garland)	Neutral/OK	
Chrysanthemum Leaves	Neutral/OK	
Cinnamon	Helpful	
Cisco	More helpful	
Cisco (smoked)	Most helpful	
Clams	More helpful	
Cloud ear fungus	Helpful	
Cloves	Neutral/OK	
Cocoa	Neutral/OK	
Coconut meat (dried)	Consume much less	
Coconut meat (raw)	Consume much less	
Coconut milk	Consume less	
Cod	Helpful	
Coffee	Neutral/OK	
Coffee (decaf)	Neutral/OK	
Coffee liqueur	Avoid	
Coffeecake	Avoid	
Cole slaw	Consume less	
Collards	Neutral/OK	
Conch	Helpful	
Consult your doctor	Most helpful	
Cookies (animal crackers)	Avoid	
Cookies (butter)	Avoid	
Cookies (chocolate chip)	Avoid	
Cookies (gingersnaps)	Avoid	
Cookies (lady fingers)	Avoid	
Cookies (molasses)	Avoid	
Cookies (oatmeal)	Avoid	
Cookies (peanut butter)	Avoid	
Cookies (shortbread)	Avoid	
Cookies (sugar)	Avoid	
Cookies (vanilla wafers)	Avoid	

Food Item or Other	Suitability for HT	Remarks (if any)
Coriander/Cilantro	Neutral/OK	
Corn	Consume less	
Corn bran	Consume less	
Corn cakes	Consume less	
Corn syrup	Consume much less	
Corned beef	Consume much less	
Cornmeal (whole-grain)	Consume much less	
Cornnuts	Consume less	
Cottonseed meal	Consume much less	
Couscous	Consume less	
Cowberries	Neutral/OK	
Cowpeas leafy tips	Neutral/OK	
Crab (Alaskan King)	More helpful	
Crab (Blue)	Helpful	
Crab (Dungeness)	More helpful	
Crab (snow)	More helpful	
Crackers (matzo)	Consume less	
Crackers (milk)	Consume much less	
Crackers (saltines)	Consume less	
Crackers (wheat)	Avoid	
Crackers (whole-wheat)	Consume much less	
Cranberries	Neutral/OK	
Cranberry juice	Consume less	
Crayfish	Helpful	
Cream	Consume less	
Cream (whipped)	Avoid	
Cream puffs/Éclair	Avoid	
Crème de menthe	Avoid	
Croaker	Consume much less	
Croissant	Avoid	
Croutons	Neutral/OK	
Cucumber with peel	Neutral/OK	
Cured meats	Consume much less	
Currants (dried)	Consume less	
Currants (raw)	Consume less	
Cusk	Helpful	
Cuttlefish	Helpful	
Dandelion Greens	Neutral/OK	
Danish pastry	Avoid	
Dates	Consume less	
Dessert toppings	Avoid	
Dill weed	Neutral/OK	
Dolphinfish (Mahi-Mahi)	More helpful	
Donuts	Avoid	
Drum	More helpful	
Duck (no skin)	Consume less	
Durian	Consume less	
Durum wheat	Neutral/OK	
Eel	Neutral/OK	
Egg (duck)	Consume much less	

Food Item or Other	Suitability for HT	Remarks (if any)
Egg (hard-boiled)	Avoid	
Egg (raw)	Avoid	
Egg rolls (veg)	Avoid	
Egg substitute	Helpful	
Egg white	Neutral/OK	
Egg yolk	Avoid	
Eggnog	Consume much less	
Eggplant	Neutral/OK	
Elderberries	Consume less	
Endive	Neutral/OK	
English muffins	Consume less	
English muffins (whole-wheat)	Consume less	
Epazote	Neutral/OK	
Excess body weight	Consume much less	
Exercise	More helpful	
Exercise - cardiovascular	More helpful	
Exercise - weight training	More helpful	
Falafel	Consume less	
Fat (beef/lamb/pork)	Consume much less	
Fat (chicken)	Avoid	
Fat (duck)	Avoid	
Fat (saturated)	Consume much less	
Fat (turkey)	Avoid	
Fat-free or low fat products	Consume less	
Fennel (Bulb)	Neutral/OK	
Fennel seeds	Neutral/OK	
Fiddlehead ferns	Helpful	
Figs	Consume less	
Figs (dried)	Consume less	
Fish oil (cod liver)	Most helpful	
Fish oil (herring)	Most helpful	
Fish oil (menhaden)	Most helpful	
Fish oil (salmon)	Most helpful	
Fish oil (sardine)	Most helpful	
Fish roe	Helpful	
Fish stock	Helpful	
Flatfish (flounder & sole)	Helpful	
Foie gras or liver pate	Avoid	
Food prep -- deep-fried	Avoid	
Food prep -- toasting	Consume less	
Frankfurter (beef & pork)	Avoid	
Frankfurter (chicken)	Avoid	
French fries	Avoid	
French toast	Avoid	
Frog legs	Consume less	
Frostings	Avoid	
Frozen yogurt	Avoid	
Fruit juice (sugared/concent.)	Consume less	
Fruit leather/rolls	Avoid	
Fruit punch	Consume less	

Food Item or Other	Suitability for HT	Remarks (if any)
Garden cress	Neutral/OK	
Garlic	More helpful	
Ginger	More helpful	
Ginger ale	Consume less	
Ginkgo nuts	Neutral/OK	
Goat meat	Consume less	
Goose	Avoid	
Gooseberries	Neutral/OK	
Granola bars	Avoid	
Grape juice	Consume less	
Grape leaves	Neutral/OK	
Grapefruit	Consume less	
Grapefruit juice	Consume less	
Grapes	Consume less	
Gravies (canned)	Neutral/OK	
Green beans	Neutral/OK	
Green onions (scallions)	Neutral/OK	
Grouper	More helpful	
Guava	Consume less	
Guggul	Helpful	
Guinea hen	Neutral/OK	
Haddock	Helpful	
Halibut	Most helpful	
Halvah (candy)	Avoid	
Hamburger	Avoid	
Hash brown potatoes	Avoid	
Hazelnuts or Filberts	Avoid	
Hearts of palm	Neutral/OK	
Herring	Most helpful	
Hickory nuts	Avoid	
Honey	Avoid	
Honeydew melon	Consume less	
Horseradish	Neutral/OK	
Hot chocolate	Consume less	
Hot dog	Avoid	
Hummus	Avoid	
Hush puppies	Avoid	
Hydrogenated vegetable oil	Avoid	
Ice cream (chocolate)	Avoid	
Ice cream (vanilla)	Avoid	
Ice cream cones	Avoid	
Jams & Preserves	Avoid	
Jellies	Avoid	
Jujube (fruit)	Consume less	
Kale	Neutral/OK	
Kelp	Neutral/OK	
Ketchup	Consume less	
Kimchi	Helpful	
Kiwi fruit	Consume less	
Kohlrabi	Neutral/OK	

Food Item or Other	Suitability for HT	Remarks (if any)
Kumquats	Consume less	
Lamb (ground)	Consume much less	
Lamb brain	Avoid	
Lamb heart	Avoid	
Lamb kidneys	Consume much less	
Lamb leg	Consume less	
Lamb liver	Consume much less	
Lamb loin	Consume much less	
Lamb ribs	Avoid	
Lamb shoulder	Consume much less	
Lamb spleen	Avoid	
Lamb tongue	Avoid	
Lambsquarters	Neutral/OK	
Lard	Avoid	
Leeks	Neutral/OK	
Lemon	Neutral/OK	
Lemonade	Consume less	
Lentils	Neutral/OK	
Lettuce (head)	Neutral/OK	
Lettuce (loose leaf)	Neutral/OK	
Lettuce (Romaine)	Neutral/OK	
Lime	Neutral/OK	
Ling	Helpful	
Lingcod	Helpful	
Litchi	Consume less	
Litchi (dried)	Consume less	
Lobster	Helpful	
Lobster (spiny)	More helpful	
Loganberry	Consume less	
Longans	Consume less	
Longans (dried)	Consume less	
Lotus root	Consume less	
Luncheon meat (beef)	Avoid	
Luncheon meat (cured beef)	Consume much less	
Luncheon meat (pork)	Avoid	
Lupin	Consume less	
Macadamia nuts	Consume less	
Macaroni	Consume less	
Mace	Neutral/OK	
Mackerel	Most helpful	
Mackerel (king)	Most helpful	
Malted drinks (nonalcoholic)	Consume less	
Mango	Consume less	
Margarine (salted)	Avoid	
Margarine (unsalted)	Avoid	
Margarine-like spreads	Avoid	
Marjoram	Neutral/OK	
Marlin	Most helpful	
Marshmallows	Avoid	
Mayonnaise	Avoid	

Food Item or Other	Suitability for HT	Remarks (if any)
Melba toast	Consume much less	
Milk (1% fat)	Consume much less	
Milk (2% fat)	Consume much less	
Milk (chocolate)	Avoid	
Milk (skim)	Consume much less	
Milk (whole)	Avoid	
Milk shakes	Consume much less	
Milkfish	More helpful	
Millet	Consume less	
Mints	Neutral/OK	
Miso	Helpful	
Molasses	Avoid	
Monkfish	Helpful	
Muffins (blueberry)	Avoid	
Muffins (corn)	Avoid	
Muffins (oat bran)	Avoid	
Muffins (wheat bran)	Avoid	
Mulberries	Consume less	
Mullet	More helpful	
Mushrooms (Chanterelle)	Helpful	
Mushrooms (Jew's ear)	Helpful	
Mushrooms (Morel)	Helpful	
Mushrooms (portabella)	Helpful	
Mushrooms (shitake)	Helpful	
Mussels	Most helpful	
Mustard	Neutral/OK	
Mustard greens	Neutral/OK	
Mustard seed	Neutral/OK	
Mustard spinach	Neutral/OK	
Nachos	Avoid	
Natal Plum (Carissa)	Neutral/OK	
Natto	Avoid	
Nectarine	Consume less	
Non-dairy creamers	Avoid	
Noodles (Chinese chow Mein)	Avoid	
Noodles (egg)	Consume less	
Noodles (Japanese)	Consume less	
Noodles (rice)	Consume less	
Nopal	Neutral/OK	
Northern pike	Helpful	
Nutmeg	Neutral/OK	
Oat bran	Neutral/OK	
Oatmeal (cereal)	Consume less	
Oats	Helpful	
Octopus	More helpful	
Oil (almonds)	Avoid	
Oil (apricot kernel)	Avoid	
Oil (avocado)	Avoid	
Oil (Babassu)	Consume much less	
Oil (canola)	Consume much less	

Food Item or Other	Suitability for HT	Remarks (if any)
Oil (Cocoa Butter)	Avoid	
Oil (coconut)	Consume much less	
Oil (corn)	Avoid	
Oil (cottonseed)	Avoid	
Oil (Cupu Assu)	Avoid	
Oil (flaxseed)	Helpful	
Oil (grape seeds)	Avoid	
Oil (hazelnut)	Avoid	
Oil (mustard)	Avoid	
Oil (oat)	Avoid	
Oil (olive)	Helpful	
Oil (palm)	Avoid	
Oil (peanut)	Avoid	
Oil (poppy seed)	Avoid	
Oil (rice bran)	Avoid	
Oil (safflower)	Avoid	
Oil (sesame)	Avoid	
Oil (Shea nut)	Consume much less	
Oil (soybean)	Avoid	
Oil (sunflower)	Avoid	
Oil (tea seed)	Avoid	
Oil (tomato seeds)	Avoid	
Oil (Ucuhuba Butter)	Avoid	
Oil (walnut)	Avoid	
Oil (wheat germ)	Avoid	
Okra	Neutral/OK	
Olives	Neutral/OK	
Omega-3 fatty acids	Most helpful	
Omega-6 fatty acid (LA)	Avoid	
Onion rings	Avoid	
Onions	Helpful	
Orange juice	Neutral/OK	
Orange roughy	Helpful	
Oranges	Consume less	
Oregano	Neutral/OK	
Oysters	More helpful	
Pancakes	Consume much less	
Pancreas	Avoid	
Papaya	Consume less	
Parsley	Neutral/OK	
Parsnips	Neutral/OK	
Passion fruit	Consume less	
Pasta	Consume less	
Pastrami (cured beef)	Consume much less	
Pastrami (turkey)	Avoid	
Peaches	Consume less	
Peaches (dried)	Consume less	
Peanut butter	Avoid	
Peanuts	Avoid	
Pears	Consume less	

Food Item or Other	Suitability for HT	Remarks (if any)
Pears (dried)	Consume less	
Peas (green)	Neutral/OK	
Peas (split)	Neutral/OK	
Peas (sugar/snap)	Neutral/OK	
Pecans	Avoid	
Pepper (black)	Neutral/OK	
Peppermint	Neutral/OK	
Pepperoni	Avoid	
Peppers (ancho)	Consume less	
Peppers (banana)	Neutral/OK	
Peppers (hot chili)	Helpful	
Peppers (hot chili, red)	Helpful	
Peppers (jalapeno)	Helpful	
Peppers (pasilla)	Neutral/OK	
Peppers (pimento)	Helpful	
Perch	Helpful	
Persimmons	Consume less	
Pheasant	Consume less	
Pheasant breast	Helpful	
Pickle (cucumber)	Neutral/OK	
Pickle (sweet)	Consume less	
Pickle relish	Neutral/OK	
Pie (apple)	Avoid	
Pie (coconut cream)	Avoid	
Pie (fried, fruit)	Avoid	
Pie (lemon meringue)	Avoid	
Pie (pecan)	Avoid	
Pie (pumpkin)	Avoid	
Pie (vanilla cream)	Avoid	
Pie crust	Avoid	
Pigeon peas	Consume less	
Pili nuts	Avoid	
Piña colada	Consume much less	
Pine nuts	Avoid	
Pineapple	Consume less	
Pineapple juice	Consume less	
Pistachio nuts	Avoid	
Pitanga	Neutral/OK	
Pizza	Avoid	
Plantains	Consume less	
Plum	Consume less	
Pokeberry shoots	Neutral/OK	
Pollock	Most helpful	
Pomegranate	Consume less	
Pomegranate juice	Consume less	
Pompano fish	More helpful	
Popcorn (air popped)	Avoid	
Popcorn (oil popped)	Avoid	
Poppy seed	Consume less	
Pork back ribs	Consume much less	

Food Item or Other	Suitability for HT	Remarks (if any)
Pork breakfast strips	Avoid	
Pork cured/ham	Consume much less	
Pork headcheese	Avoid	
Pork heart	Avoid	
Pork kidneys	Avoid	
Pork leg/ham	Consume much less	
Pork liver	Consume much less	
Pork liver cheese	Avoid	
Pork loin/sirloin	Consume less	
Pork lungs	Avoid	
Pork ribs	Avoid	
Pork shoulder	Avoid	
Pork skins	Avoid	
Pork spare ribs	Avoid	
Pork spleen	Avoid	
Potato	Neutral/OK	
Potato chips	Avoid	
Potato pancakes	Avoid	
Potato salad	Avoid	
Potato sticks	Avoid	
Potatoes w/skin	Consume less	
Pout	Helpful	
Pretzels	Consume less	
Prune juice	Consume less	
Prunes (dried)	Consume less	
Pudding	Avoid	
Puff pastry	Avoid	
Pumelo (Shaddock)	Neutral/OK	
Pumpkin	Neutral/OK	
Pumpkin flowers	Neutral/OK	
Pumpkinseed sunfish	Helpful	
Purslane	Neutral/OK	
Quail	Consume much less	
Quail breast	Helpful	
Quince	Consume less	
Quinoa	Consume less	
Rabbit meat	Consume less	
Radishes	Neutral/OK	
Raisins	Consume less	
Raspberries	Neutral/OK	
Red Bull (drink)	Helpful	
Rhubarb	Neutral/OK	
Rice (brown)	Consume less	
Rice (white)	Neutral/OK	
Rice (wild)	Consume less	
Rice bran	Helpful	
Rice cakes (Brown rice)	Helpful	
Rockfish	Helpful	
Rolls (French)	Consume less	
Rolls (hamburger/hot dog)	Consume less	

Food Item or Other	Suitability for HT	Remarks (if any)
Rolls (Kaiser)	Consume much less	
Rolls (whole-wheat dinner)	Avoid	
Rosemary (fresh)	Neutral/OK	
Rowal	Consume less	
Rutabaga	Neutral/OK	
Rye grain	Consume less	
Sablefish	Most helpful	
Saccharine (NutraSweet)	Consume less	
Saffron	Neutral/OK	
Sage	Neutral/OK	
Salad dressing (1000 Island)	Avoid	
Salad dressing (Blue/Roquefort)	Avoid	
Salad dressing (French)	Avoid	
Salad dressing (Italian)	Avoid	
Salami (various)	Avoid	
Salmon (pink)	Most helpful	
Salmon (smoked, Lox)	Most helpful	
Salt (table)	Neutral/OK	
Sardines	Neutral/OK	
Sauce (cheese)	Neutral/OK	
Sauce (fish)	Neutral/OK	
Sauce (Hoisin)	Consume less	
Sauce (oyster)	Neutral/OK	
Sauce (pepper or hot)	Neutral/OK	
Sauce (sofrito)	Neutral/OK	
Sauce (tomato)	Neutral/OK	
Sauerkraut	Neutral/OK	
Sausage (blood)	Avoid	
Sausage (liver)	Avoid	
Sausage (meatless)	Avoid	
Sausage (smoked)	Avoid	
Scallops	Helpful	
Scup	Helpful	
Seatrout	More helpful	
Seeds (breadnut tree)	Neutral/OK	
Seeds (chia)	Helpful	
Seeds (cottonseed)	Avoid	
Seeds (flaxseed)	Helpful	
Seeds (pumpkin/squash)	Avoid	
Seeds (safflower)	Avoid	
Seeds (sesame)	Avoid	
Seeds (sunflower)	Avoid	
Seeds (watermelon)	Avoid	
Semolina	Neutral/OK	
Sesbania Flower	Neutral/OK	
Shad	More helpful	
Shallots	Consume less	
Shark	Neutral/OK	
Sheepshead	Helpful	
Sherbet	Avoid	

Food Item or Other	Suitability for HT	Remarks (if any)
Shrimp	Helpful	
Smelt	Most helpful	
Smoking/Tobacco	Consume much less	
Snail	Helpful	
Snapper	More helpful	
Soft (carbonated) drinks	Consume much less	
Sorghum grain	Neutral/OK	
Soup (beef barley)	Consume less	
Soup (chicken noodle)	Consume less	
Soup (clam chowder)	Helpful	
Soup (veg/beef)	Consume less	
Sour cream	Consume much less	
Soy milk	Consume less	
Soy sauce	Consume much less	
Soybeans (dried)	More helpful	
Soybeans (green)	Consume less	
Spaghetti	Consume less	
Spaghetti (spinach)	Neutral/OK	
Spaghetti (whole-wheat)	Consume less	
Spearmint (fresh)	Neutral/OK	
Spelt	Consume less	
Spinach	Neutral/OK	
Sports drinks	Consume less	
Spot	Most helpful	
Squab (pigeon)	Consume much less	
Squash (Acorn)	Neutral/OK	
Squash (Butternut)	Neutral/OK	
Squash (Hubbard)	Neutral/OK	
Squash (Spaghetti)	Neutral/OK	
Squid (Calamari)	Neutral/OK	
Starfruit	Neutral/OK	
Strawberries	Neutral/OK	
Sturgeon	Most helpful	
Succotash	Neutral/OK	
Sucker	Most helpful	
Sugar (brown)	Consume much less	
Sugar (maple)	Consume less	
Sugar (refined)	Consume less	
Sugar (table, powder)	Consume much less	
Sugar (total)	Consume less	
Surimi	More helpful	
Sweet potatoes	Consume less	
Sweet potatoes leaves	Neutral/OK	
Sweet rolls	Avoid	
Swiss chard	Neutral/OK	
Swordfish	Most helpful	
Syrup (chocolate)	Avoid	
Syrup (malt)	Consume much less	
Syrup (maple)	Avoid	
Syrup (sorghum)	Avoid	

Food Item or Other	Suitability for HT	Remarks (if any)
Syrup (table blends)	Avoid	
Tabasco sauce	Neutral/OK	
Taco shells	Avoid	
Tahini	Avoid	
Tamarind	Consume much less	
Tangerines	Consume less	
Tapioca pearls	Consume less	
Taro	Consume less	
Taro (Tahitian)	Neutral/OK	
Taro chips	Avoid	
Taro leaves	Helpful	
Tarragon	Neutral/OK	
Tea (green)	Helpful	
Tea (herbal)	Neutral/OK	
Tea (plain)	Neutral/OK	
Tempeh	Consume less	
Teriyaki sauce	Avoid	
Thyme (fresh)	Neutral/OK	
Tilapia	More helpful	
Tilefish	Most helpful	
Toasted bread	Consume less	
Tofu	Consume less	
Tofu (fried)	Consume much less	
Tomato juice	Neutral/OK	
Tomato paste	Neutral/OK	
Tomatoes	Neutral/OK	
Tomatoes (sun-dried)	Helpful	
Tonic water	Consume less	
Tortilla chips	Avoid	
Tortillas (corn)	Consume much less	
Trans fatty acids	Avoid	
Triticale	Helpful	
Trout	Most helpful	
Tuna (blue fin)	Most helpful	
Tuna (canned)	Helpful	
Tuna (yellowfin)	Most helpful	
Turbot	Helpful	
Turkey breast	Neutral/OK	
Turkey dark meat	Neutral/OK	
Turkey giblets	Avoid	
Turkey heart	Avoid	
Turkey liver	Consume much less	
Turkey skins	Avoid	
Turmeric	Neutral/OK	
Turnip greens	Neutral/OK	
Turnips	Neutral/OK	
Veal heart	Avoid	
Veal kidneys	Avoid	
Veal liver	Consume much less	
Veal loin	Helpful	

Food Item or Other	Suitability for HT	Remarks (if any)
Veal lungs	Avoid	
Veal shank	Helpful	
Veal shoulder	Neutral/OK	
Veal spleen	Avoid	
Veal thymus	Avoid	
Veal tongue	Avoid	
Vegetable shortening	Avoid	
Venison	Neutral/OK	
Vine spinach (Basella)	Neutral/OK	
Vinegar	Neutral/OK	
Vitamin B-3 (Niacin)	More helpful; in nicotinic acid form, not recommended as supplement or drug	
Vitamin B-5 (Pantothenic Acid)	Helpful	For HT, in pantethine form
Waffles	Avoid	
Walk, wheel, or jog	More helpful	
Walleye	More helpful	
Walnuts	Avoid	
Walnuts (black)	Avoid	
Wasabi root	Neutral/OK	
Water	Neutral/OK	
Watercress	Neutral/OK	
Watermelon	Consume less	
Wheat	Consume less	
Wheat bran	Helpful	
Wheat germ	Consume less	
Whelk	Neutral/OK	
Whey (sweet)	Consume less	
Whiskey	Consume less	
White fish	Most helpful	
White fish (smoked)	More helpful	
Whiting	More helpful	
Whole-wheat	Neutral/OK	
Wild fish and free range animals	More helpful	
Wine (red)	Consume less	
Wine (white)	Consume less	
Winged beans leaves	Helpful	
Wolffish	Most helpful	
Yam	Consume less	
Yellowtail	More helpful	
Yogurt	Consume less	
Zucchini	Neutral/OK	

High Cholesterol (& HT)

Cholesterol is a fat-like substance found in every cell of your body. Your body needs cholesterol to function properly, and it normally produces the amount of cholesterol that it requires. However, many foods that you consume can also result in increase in the level of cholesterol in your body -- in your blood in particular. There is usually no symptom for high cholesterol, but it can be discovered through a routine blood test.

High levels of cholesterol in your blood can result in build-up of what is known as plaque in your arteries. Plaque can narrow or block your arteries. Since arteries carry blood from your heart to the rest of your body, high level of cholesterol can result in heart disease and damage your cardiovascular system.

Cholesterol exists in two forms in your blood known as: LDL and HDL. LDL is called bad cholesterol because it leads to build up of plaque in your arteries. HDL is called good cholesterol because it removes and carries cholesterol away and delivers it to your liver where it gets eliminated from your body.

Your LDL is considered too high if it is greater than 160 milligram per deciliter. Your HDL is considered too low if it is less than 40 mg/dl. Your total cholesterol is considered too high if it is greater than 240 mg/dl, and is considered desirable if it is less than 200 mg/dl.

You are likely to have high cholesterol if you consume too much animal fat and trans fatty acids, you are not physically active, you are overweight, and there is a history of the same in your family. Your cholesterol levels tend to rise as you get older.

Choose these for   High Cholesterol & HT

Top 5 items to choose:

> ### Fish & Mussels; Mushrooms; Garlic; Ginger; Soybeans; ... and Exercise

Food items and actions that could improve your health (within a food group, most helpful items are listed first):

Meat, Fish & Poultry (2+ fish meals per week)

Anchovy; Bluefish; Cisco (smoked); Mackerel (king); Marlin; Spot; Sturgeon; Swordfish; Trout; Tuna (blue fin); White fish; Sablefish; Tilefish; Bass (striped); Tuna (yellowfin); Halibut; Wolffish; Pollock; Sucker; Smelt; Bass (seabass); Bass (freshwater); Drum; Whiting; Mackerel; Salmon (pink); Herring; Milkfish; Yellowtail; Mullet; Cisco; Caviar; Salmon (smoked, Lox); Surimi; Mussels; Tilapia; Shad; Snapper; Pompano fish; Butterfish; Scup; Flatfish (flounder & sole); Cusk; Seatrout; Walleye; Catfish; Lingcod; Rockfish; White fish (smoked); Grouper; Northern pike; Dolphinfish (Mahi-Mahi); Tuna (canned); Carp; Haddock; Cod; Burbot; Oysters; Monkfish; Sheepshead; Perch; Crab (Dungeness); Shark; Ling; Pumpkinseed sunfish; Turbot; Lobster (spiny); Fish roe; Crab (snow); Pout; Chicken breast (no skin); Orange roughy; Crab (Alaskan King); Pheasant breast; Sardines; Clams; Veal loin; Conch; Octopus; Scallops; Beef filet mignon; Quail breast; Snail;

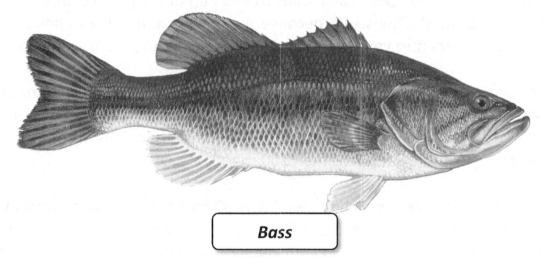

Bass

Eggs, Beans, Nuts and Seeds

Soybeans (dried); Peas (sugar/snap); Peas (green); Lentils; Peas (split); Various Beans; Pigeon peas; Black-eyed peas; Seeds: chia, flaxseed; Macadamia nuts; Lupin; Alfalfa sprouts; Chickpeas; Ginkgo nuts; Egg substitute; Egg white; Soy milk; Breadfruit seeds; Seeds (breadnut tree);

Fruits & Juices

Blackberries; Raspberries; Cranberries; Guava; Passion fruit; Currants (raw); Other Berries; Rhubarb; Plum; Watermelon; Apricots; Cantaloupe; Grapefruit; Pomegranate; Peaches; Lemon; Lime; Starfruit; Papaya; Mango; Abiyuch; Kumquats; Rowal; Cranberry juice; Durian; Kiwi fruit; Apples (eat with skin); Acerola; Natal Plum (Carissa); Olives; Pitanga; Pumelo (Shaddock); Nectarine; Apricots (dried); Currants (dried); Grapes; Grapefruit juice; Honeydew melon; Jujube (fruit); Pineapple; Pineapple juice; Tangerines; Banana; Dried Fruits; Breadfruit; Cherries; Grape juice; Persimmons; Pomegranate juice; Figs; Plantains; Tamarind; Quince; Raisins; Blueberries; Oranges; Dates; Litchi; Prune juice; Longans; Avocado; Pears; **Avoid sugared or made from concentrate juices;**

Vegetables

Mushrooms (shitake); **Garlic**; **Mushrooms: Chanterelle, portabella**; **Cloud ear fungus**; **Chicory greens**; **Taro leaves**; **Peppers (pimento)**; **Tomatoes (sun-dried)**; **Broccoli**; **Endive**; **Onions**; Cabbage (savoy); Sweet potatoes leaves; Tomato juice; Grape leaves; Peppers (jalapeno); Dandelion Greens; Collards; Mustard greens; Turnip greens; Broccoli (Chinese); Cabbage (red); Carrots; Chrysanthemum (Garland); Squash (Butternut); Squash (Hubbard); Tomatoes; Sweet potatoes; Cabbage (green); Beet greens; Winged beans leaves; Spinach; Arugula; Bok choy; Garden cress; Kale; Various Lettuce; Pokeberry shoots; Pumpkin; Watercress; Other Mushrooms; Brussels sprouts; Green onions (scallions); Other Peppers; Swiss chard; Asparagus; Arrowroot; Squash (Acorn); Green beans; Okra; Zucchini; Fiddlehead ferns; Artichoke; Leeks; Balsam pear; Cauliflower; Kohlrabi; Parsnips; Other vegetables;

Breads, Grains, Cereals, Pasta

Barley; Oat bran (3 grams daily); Triticale; Corn bran; Rice cakes (Brown rice); English muffins (whole-wheat); Rye grain; Rice bran; Durum wheat; Sorghum grain Whole-wheat; Wheat bran; Oatmeal (cereal); Oats; Bread (whole-wheat); Bulgur; Spaghetti (whole-wheat); Corn; Buckwheat; Quinoa; Spelt; Millet; Rice (brown); Rice (wild); Spaghetti (spinach);

Dairy Products, Fats & Oils

Fish oil (salmon); **Fish oil (cod liver)**; **Oil (olive; extra virgin)**; Other Fish oil; Oil (flaxseed); Yogurt;

Desserts, Snacks, Beverages

Red Bull (drink); Tea (green; Do not brew or drink tea scolding hot); Tea (plain); Water;

Herbs & Spices, Prepared & Fast Foods

Ginger; Soup (clam chowder); Cayenne (red) pepper; Cinnamon; Parsley; Turmeric; Fish stock; Soup (minestrone); Tomato paste; Saffron; Miso; Thyme (fresh); Coriander/Cilantro; Soup (vegetable); Soup (tomato); Basil (fresh); Cocoa; Succotash;

Alternative Therapies & Miscellaneous

Exercise (including cardiovascular, weight training, walk, wheel, or jog); **Wild fish and free range animals**; Glucomannan;

Key Nutrients & Herbal Meds

Omega-3 fatty acids; **Vitamin B-3 (Niacin; in nicotinic acid form, not recommended as supplement or drug)**; **Psyllium**; Celery seed; Fenugreek seeds; Fiber (soluble fiber); Guggul; Vitamin B-5 (Pantothenic Acid; in pantethine form); Yucca; Fat (monounsaturated; limit to 20% of total daily calories);

Do not choose these for   High Cholesterol & HT

Top 5 items to avoid:

> Margarine; Sweets; Luncheon (processed) Meats;
> Hydrogenated Vegetable Oil & Shortening; Cheese;

Avoid or consume much less of the following (within a food group, most harmful items are listed first):

Meat, Fish & Poultry

Bacon; Beef (cured brkfst strips); Beef jerky sticks; Beef tongue; Salami; Bologna; Chicken heart; Chicken skin; Chorizo; Frankfurters; Lamb tongue; Luncheon meats; Organ Meats; Pepperoni; Pork breakfast strips; Pork ribs; Pork skins; Pork spare ribs; Salami; Sausages; Turkey skins; Pastrami; Beef chuck/brisket; Goose; Pork; Lamb ribs; Corned beef; Beef (ground); Cured meats; Chicken wings; Chicken dark meat; Beef; Lamb; Beaver meat; Squab (pigeon); Bear meat; Quail; Bison/buffalo meat; Boar meat; Cuttlefish; Duck (no skin); Shrimp; Frog legs; Goat meat; Abalone; Squid (Calamari); Whelk; Rabbit meat; Venison; Beef top sirloin; Turkey dark meat; Eel; Guinea hen; Beef rib eye; Turkey breast;

Instead **choose**: Lobster; Crab (Blue); Veal shank; Pheasant; Veal shoulder; Crayfish; Croaker;

Eggs, Beans, Nuts and Seeds

Egg yolk; Seeds: cottonseed, watermelon; Egg (hard-boiled); Seeds (pumpkin/squash); Coconut meat (dried); Egg (raw); Seeds (safflower); Pili nuts; Brazil nuts; Butternuts; Pine nuts; Coconut meat (raw); Hickory nuts; Egg (duck); Cashew nuts; Beechnuts; Seeds (sunflower); Coconut milk; Walnuts (black); Pistachio nuts; Pecans; Acorns; Peanuts; Seeds (sesame); Hazelnuts or Filberts; Almonds; Soybeans (green);

Instead **choose**: Cornnuts; Walnuts; Chestnuts;

Breads, Grains, Cereals, Pasta

Croissant; Danish pastry; Donuts; Muffins (blueberry); Muffins (oat bran); Sweet rolls; Waffles; Cereal (granola); Bread (cornbread); Granola bars; Crackers (wheat); Biscuits; Muffins (wheat bran); Bread (banana); Crackers (milk); Muffins (corn); Cereals; Rolls (Kaiser); Cereal (wheat germ); Bread sticks; Noodles (Chinese chow Mein); Crackers (whole-wheat); Rolls (whole-wheat dinner); Crackers (saltines); Melba toast; Wheat germ; Rolls (hamburger/hot dog); Bagels; Cereals: rice crisps, cream of wheat; Noodles (egg); Rolls (French); Tortillas (corn); Bread (white); Bread (Italian); Pasta; English muffins; Bread (pumpernickel); Crackers (matzo); Cereals: shredded wheat, raisin bran;

Instead **choose**: Amaranth; Breads: wheat germ, French/Sourdough, oat bran; Cereals: corn flakes, whole-wheat, bran flakes; Croutons; Semolina; Couscous; Other Noodles; Wheat; Rice (white); Spaghetti;

Dairy Products, Fats & Oils

Margarine (use soft or liquid vegetable oils instead); **Various Cheese; Cheese spread; Cream (whipped); Fat (chicken, duck, turkey); Hydrogenated vegetable oil; Lard; Vegetable shortening; Oil (Ucuhuba Butter); Non-dairy creamers; Oil (cottonseed); Margarine-like spreads; Various Oils; Fat (beef/lamb/pork); Butter; Milk (chocolate); Sour cream; Milk (whole); Milk (skim);** Oil (almonds); Milk (1% fat); Buttermilk; Milk (2% fat); Oils: hazelnut, safflower, canola; Cream; Whey (sweet); Cheese (Cottage);

Desserts, Snacks, Beverages

Coffeecake; After-dinner mints; Brownies; Cakes; Candies (caramel); Carob (candy); Cheesecake; Chocolate mousse; Cookies; Cream puffs/Éclair; Dessert toppings; Halvah (candy); Ice creams; Pies; Potato sticks; Puff pastry; Taro chips; Fruit leather/rolls; Candies; Frostings; Pie crust; Chewing gum; Marshmallows; Pudding; Tortilla chips; Frozen yogurt; Sherbet; Jams & Preserves; Jellies; Peanut butter; Ice cream cones; Chocolate (sweet); Pancakes; Pie (pumpkin); Coffee liqueur; Crème de menthe; Honey; Popcorn (oil popped); Eggnog; Molasses; Potato chips; Milk shakes; Chocolate (dark); Pretzels; Piña colada; Applesauce; Soft (carbonated) drinks; Fruit punch; Lemonade; Ginger ale; Hot chocolate; Tonic water; Sports drinks; Malted drinks (nonalcoholic); 80+ proof distilled alc. bev.; Whiskey; Popcorn (air popped); Wine (white);

Instead *choose*: Wine (red); Coffee; Coffee (decaf); Orange juice; Tea (herbal); Beer;

Herbs & Spices, Prepared & Fast Foods

Breaded shrimp; Cheeseburger; Foie gras or liver pate; French toast; Hush puppies; Nachos; Onion rings; Pizza; Potato pancakes; Salad dressings; Potato salad; Taco shells; Hot dog; Teriyaki sauce; Syrup (chocolate); Hamburger; Soy sauce; Hash brown potatoes; Sausage (meatless); Syrup (maple); Natto; Chicken Nuggets; Cottonseed meal; Syrup (sorghum); Sugar (table, powder); Syrup (table blends); French fries; Mayonnaise; Hummus; Sugar (brown); Egg rolls (veg); Barbecue sauce; Sauces; Tofu (fried); Pickle (sweet); Tahini; Beef broth & stock; Chicken broth; Soup (chicken noodle); Ketchup; Poppy seed; Macaroni; Salt (table); Corn cakes; Sugar (maple); Chicken stock; Soup (beef barley); Falafel; Tofu; Syrup (malt); Sauce (pepper or hot); Tabasco sauce; Soup (veg/beef);

Instead *choose*: Tempeh; Cornmeal (whole-grain); Pepper (black); Herbs & Spices; Balsamic vinegar; Gravies; Horseradish; Pickle; Vinegar; Kimchi; Sauce (tomato); Cole slaw; Mustard; Sauerkraut; Capers;

Alternative Therapies & Miscellaneous

Deep-fried Foods; Smoking/Tobacco; Baking using butter; Excess body weight; 2+ alcoholic drinks/day; Cheese made w/whole milk; Corn syrup; Canned foods; Artificial sweeteners; Processed or Refined foods;

Key Nutrients & Herbal Meds

Trans fatty acids; Fat, saturated (limit to 7% of daily calories); Omega-6 fatty acid (LA); Cholesterol (Limit to less than 200 mg per day); Sugar (refined);

High Blood Pressure (& HT)

High blood pressure (HBP), also known as Hypertension, is a serious condition and can lead to other health issues such as heart attack, stroke and kidney failure.

Your blood pressure is an indication of how hard your heart has to work to pump blood through your arteries and how much resistance to blood flow exists in your arteries. It is highest when your heart beats, pumping the blood (systolic pressure). And it is the lowest between beats (diastolic pressure).

The blood pressure is often shown in form of a ratio, Systolic/Diastolic pressure, and measured in millimeters of mercury. Your blood pressure is considered normal if the Systolic number is less than 120 and Diastolic number is lower than 80. For example, if your blood pressure numbers are 115/79, you are fine. But if your top number is 140 or higher, or your bottom number is 90 or higher then you have HBP. If your numbers are in between normal and high, then you are likely to end up with HBP unless you take some action to prevent it.

There is no clear cause for HBP among adults. But there are some medical conditions (e.g., kidney problems, sleep apnea), certain medications (e.g., birth control pills) and use of some illegal drugs (e.g., cocaine) that can cause the blood pressure to rise.

You are more likely to develop HBP if you are: an over 55 man, an over 45 woman, black, overweight, physically inactive, under a lot of stress, smoke, drink too much alcohol, eat too much salt/sodium, do not eat enough potassium or Vitamin D, or have a family history of HBP.

Choose these for High Blood Pressure & HT

Top 5 items to consume:

Fish; Fish Oil; Soybeans; Garlic & Mushrooms; Shellfish; & Exercise;

Food items and actions that could improve your health (within a food group, most helpful items are listed first):

Meat, Fish & Poultry

Marlin; Salmon (pink); Swordfish; White fish; Trout; Tuna (blue fin); Spot; Mackerel; Herring; Sturgeon; Tilefish; Bluefish; Halibut; Cisco (smoked); Pollock; Bass (seabass); Tuna (yellowfin); Sablefish; Bass (freshwater); Bass (striped); Pompano fish; Smelt; Whiting; Mackerel (king); Sucker; Wolffish; Mullet; Snapper; Drum; Caviar; Shad; Mussels; Catfish; Walleye; Oysters; Carp; Anchovy; Seatrout; Cisco; Crab (Dungeness); Snail; Surimi; Octopus; Dolphinfish (Mahi-Mahi); Yellowtail; Rockfish; Grouper; Perch; Milkfish; Burbot; Lingcod; Tilapia; Lobster (spiny); Conch; Cusk; Whelk; Ling; Butterfish; Pumpkinseed sunfish; Scup; Sheepshead; Flatfish (flounder & sole); Northern pike; Fish roe; Monkfish; White fish (smoked); Pout; Chicken breast (no skin); Cuttlefish; Salmon (smoked, Lox); Haddock; Cod; Crab (Alaskan King); Orange roughy; Eel; Sardines; Crab (snow); Crayfish; Clams; Turbot; Lobster; Beef filet mignon; Quail breast; Crab (Blue); Veal loin; Pheasant breast; Veal shank; Scallops; Caribou meat; Squid (Calamari); Shark;

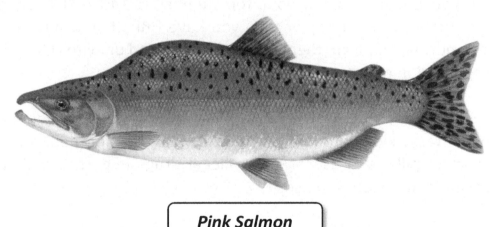

Pink Salmon

Eggs, Beans, Nuts and Seeds

Soybeans (dried); Seeds (chia); Beans: moth beans, hyacinth; Seeds (flaxseed); Alfalfa sprouts; Beans: mung, yardlong, Great northern; Lentils; Seeds (breadnut tree); Peas (green); Pigeon peas; Other Beans; Peas (sugar/snap); Peas (split); Black-eyed peas; Lupin;

Fruits & Juices

Guava; Olives; Durian; Passion fruit; Raisins; Watermelon; Blueberries; Natal Plum (Carissa); Orange juice; Plantains; Abiyuch; Breadfruit; Lemon; Lime; Starfruit; Prunes (dried); Cantaloupe; Jujube (fruit); Papaya; Tamarind; Apple juice; Grapefruit juice; Acerola; Pitanga; Pumelo (Shaddock); Persimmons; Raspberries; Kumquats; Peaches; Banana (dried); Prune juice; Honeydew melon; Nectarine; Pineapple; Pineapple juice; Plum; Banana; Rowal; Pomegranate juice; Blackberries; Strawberries; Pomegranate; Dried Fruits; Currants (raw); Grapefruit; Pears; Berries; Dates; Cherries; Quince; Longans; Apricots; Grapes; Apples; Tangerines; Grape juice; Oranges; **Avoid sugared or made from concentrate juices;**

Vegetables

Garlic; **Mushrooms: Chanterelle, Shitake, Morel**; **Taro leaves**; **Tomatoes (sun-dried)**; **Artichoke**; **Arrowroot; Onions (for HBP, 2-5 oz. of fresh onion daily, or 1 tsp. onion juice 3-4 times a day);** Amaranth leaves; Balsam pear leafy tips; Epazote; Lambsquarters; Mustard spinach; Peppers (pasilla); Taro (Tahitian); Garden cress; Sweet potatoes leaves; Mushrooms (portabella); Cloud ear fungus; Grape leaves; Winged beans leaves; Vine spinach (Basella); Arrowhead; Yam; Chrysanthemum (Garland); Chrysanthemum Leaves; Cowpeas leafy tips; Kelp; Arugula; Borage; Nopal; Purslane; Peppers; Turnips; Broccoli (Chinese); Fennel (Bulb); Fiddlehead ferns; Cauliflower; Mushrooms (Jew's ear); Shallots; Taro; Bok choy; Chicory greens; Squash (Acorn); Cucumber with peel; Kohlrabi; Balsam pear; Green onions (scallions); Lotus root; Carrots; Broccoli; Celtuce; Cabbage (savoy); Brussels sprouts; Cabbage (green); Tomato juice; Rutabaga; Radishes; Bell peppers (red); Cabbage (red); Various Lettuce; Pokeberry shoots; Pumpkin flowers; Sesbania Flower; Wasabi root; Watercress; Squash (Hubbard); Artichoke (Jerusalem); Squash (Butternut); Potatoes w/skin; Potato; Spinach; Celery; Tomatoes; Zucchini; Pumpkin; Hearts of palm; Mustard greens; Kale; Eggplant; Bell peppers (green); Beet greens; Squash (Spaghetti); Dandelion Greens; Okra; Green beans; Sweet potatoes; Asparagus;

Breads, Grains, Cereals, Pasta

Rice bran; Triticale; Quinoa; Sorghum grain; Millet; Oats; Rice (wild); Rye grain; Rice cakes (Brown rice); English muffins (whole-wheat); Spelt; Bread (whole-wheat); Corn; Bulgur; Durum wheat; Corn bran; Wheat bran; Buckwheat; Oatmeal (cereal); Whole-wheat; Spaghetti (spinach);

Dairy Products, Fats & Oils

Fish oil (cod liver); **Various Fish oil**; Oil (flaxseed); Cheese (Cottage); Yogurt; Fat-free or low fat products;

Desserts, Snacks, Beverages

Water; Coffee (decaf);

Herbs & Spices, Fast Foods, Prepared Foods

Cinnamon (especially effective with pre-diabetic & high blood pressure); Ginger; Tofu; Fish stock; Succotash; Cottonseed meal; Cayenne (red) pepper; Cocoa; Fennel seeds; Tempeh; Pickle (cucumber); Corn salad; Cornmeal (whole-grain); Balsamic vinegar; Vinegar;

Alternative Therapies & Miscellaneous

Exercise (including cardiovascular, weight training, walk, wheel, or jog); **DASH diet**; Organically grown foods; Wild fish and free range animals; Fresh (uncooked) fruits/veg's; Meditation; Pray, practice your religion; Sleep 6-8 hours regularly; Tai Chi; Yoga (certain postures like inversion poses must be avoided); Salt-free or low-salt foods; Fat-free or low fat products;

Key Nutrients & Herbal Meds

Omega-3 fatty acids; **Hawthorn (In berries form or tea from dried leaves and flowers, do not take with other heart medications)**; Anise seed; Barberry; Calcium; Celery seed; Ginseng (Siberian); Magnesium; Potassium; Vitamin B-3 (Niacin; in nicotinic acid form, not recommended as supplement or drug); Yucca;

Do not choose these for High Blood Pressure & HT

Top 5 items to avoid:

Chocolate; Sweets; Luncheon (processed) Meats;
Hydrogenated Vegetable Oils; Cheese; & Excess
Body Weight;

Avoid or consume much less of the following (within a food group, most harmful items are listed first):

Meat, Fish & Poultry

Bacon; Beef jerky sticks; Salami; Chorizo; Frankfurters; Luncheon meats; Pepperoni; Pork breakfast strips; Pork skins; Sausages; Bologna; Pork liver cheese; Pastrami; Turkey skins; Chicken skin; Pork headcheese; Corned beef; Beef (cured dried); Beef & Lamb tongue; Pork ribs; Pancreas; Lamb ribs; Cured meats; Pork spare ribs; Beef chuck/brisket; Goose; Chicken wings; Organ Meats; Pork cured/ham; Beef ribs; Pork shoulder; Chicken dark meat; Pork; Lamb; Beef; Quail; Squab (pigeon); Croaker; Bison/buffalo meat; Game meat; Abalone; Duck (no skin); Frog legs;

Instead choose: Turkey breast; Venison; Veal shoulder; Shrimp; Rabbit meat; Guinea hen; Pheasant; Canned Tuna; Goat meat; Beef round steak or rib eye; Turkey dark meat;

Eggs, Beans, Nuts and Seeds

Pili nuts; Butternuts; Hickory nuts; Pine nuts; Beechnuts; Pecans; Peanuts; Coconut meat (dried); Egg yolk; Acorns; Walnuts (black); Walnuts; Brazil nuts; Soy milk; Egg (hard-boiled); Cashew nuts; Egg (raw); Seeds (sesame); Coconut meat (raw); Almonds; Seeds: pumpkin/squash, safflower, watermelon, sunflower; Hazelnuts or Filberts; Egg (duck); Cornnuts; Coconut milk; Chestnuts; Seeds (cottonseed); Macadamia nuts; Breadfruit seeds; Pistachio nuts; Ginkgo nuts;

Instead choose: Beans; black, baked, navy; Egg substitute; Chickpeas; Soybeans (green);

Fruits & Juices

Figs; Figs (dried); Gooseberries; Cranberry juice; Cranberries; **Avoid sugared or made from concentrate juices;**

Instead choose: Kiwi fruit; Mango; Avocado; Litchi; Elderberries; Apricots (dried); Rhubarb;

Vegetables

Leeks;

Instead choose: Parsnips; Collards; Turnip greens; Endive; Beets; Swiss chard;

Breads, Grains, Cereals, Pasta

Croissant; **Danish pastry**; **Donuts**; **Muffins (blueberry)**; **Sweet rolls**; **Cereal (granola)**; **Biscuits**; **Crackers (wheat)**; **Bread sticks**; **Waffles**; **Bread (banana)**; **Granola bars**; **Rolls (Kaiser)**; **Muffins (wheat bran)**; **Noodles (Chinese chow Mein)**; **Bread (cornbread)**; **Crackers (milk)**; **Melba toast**; **Crackers (saltines)**; **Muffins (corn)**; **Rolls (French)**; **Rolls (hamburger/hot dog)**; **Crackers (whole-wheat)**; **Bread (Italian)**; Wheat germ; Bagels; Bread (pumpernickel); English muffins; Various Cereals; Muffins (oat bran); Toasted bread; Rolls (whole-wheat dinner); Crackers (matzo); Tortillas (corn); Bread (white); Noodles (egg); Bread (French/Sourdough); Bread (oat bran); Wheat; Couscous; Pasta; Spaghetti; Bread (wheat germ); Cereal (shredded wheat); Noodles (rice); Semolina;

Instead _choose_: Barley; Spaghetti (whole-wheat); Cereal (whole-wheat); Rice (brown); Oat bran; Noodles (Japanese); Rice (white); Amaranth;

Dairy Products, Fats & Oils

Non-dairy creamers; **Hydrogenated vegetable oil**; **Margarine**; **Oil (wheat germ)**; **Cheese (Brie)**; **Oil (cottonseed)**; **Margarine-like spreads**; **Fat (chicken, duck, turkey)**; **Lard**; **Oils: corn, palm, poppy seed, sesame, tea seed, tomato seeds**; **Vegetable shortening**; **Other Oils**; **Milk (chocolate)**; **Cream (whipped)**; **Cheese (Feta)**; **Cheese spread**; **Cheese (Camembert)**; **Cheese (Roquefort)**; **Butter (salted)**; **Various Cheese**; **Butter (unsalted)**; **Fat (beef/lamb/pork)**; Oil (canola); Cheese (Port de salut); Cheese (Cheddar); Milk (whole); Cheese (Ricotta); Cheese (Gruyere); Sour cream; Cheese (Swiss); Milk (skim); Cheese (Gjetost); Milk (1% fat); Milk (2% fat); Whey (sweet);

Instead _choose_: Buttermilk; Oil (olive); Cream;

Desserts, Snacks, Beverages

Pie (vanilla cream); **Brownies**; **Cakes**; **Candies (peanut brittle)**; **Cheesecake**; **Chocolate mousse**; **Coffee liqueur**; **Coffeecake**; **Cookies**; **Cream puffs/Éclair**; **Ice cream (chocolate)**; **Peanut butter**; **Pie (apple)**; **Pie (fried, fruit)**; **Pie crust**; **Puff pastry**; **Ice cream cones**; **Pie (pecan)**; **Dessert toppings**; **Pies**; **Frostings**; **Chocolate (sweet)**; **Pudding**; **Fruit leather/rolls**; **Crème de menthe**; **After-dinner mints**; **Potato sticks**; **Candies (caramel)**; **Ice cream (vanilla)**; **Popcorn (oil popped)**; **Candies**; **Chewing gum**; **Tortilla chips**; **Sherbet**; **Jams & Preserves**; **Potato chips**; **Taro chips**; **Pretzels**; **Marshmallows**; **Halvah (candy)**; **Pancakes**; **Frozen yogurt**; **Jellies**; **Hot chocolate**; **Honey**; **Piña colada**; Milk shakes; Fruit punch; Eggnog; Applesauce; Soft (carbonated) drinks; 80+ proof distilled alc. bev.; Lemonade; Ginger ale; Whiskey; Tonic water; Malted drinks (nonalcoholic); Red Bull (drink); Tea (plain); Sports drinks; Coffee; Chocolate (dark); Wine (white); Candies (sesame crunch); Beer;

Instead _choose_: Popcorn (air popped); Wine (red, with dinner); Molasses; Tea (green); Tea (herbal);

Herbs & Spices, Fast Foods, Prepared Foods

Foie gras or liver pate; **Onion rings**; **Breaded shrimp**; **Potato salad**; **Pizza**; **Salad dressings**; **Syrup (chocolate)**; **Hot dog**; **Teriyaki sauce**; **Sausage (meatless)**; **Nachos**; **Hash brown potatoes**; **Cheeseburger**; **Soy sauce**; **French toast**; **Hush puppies**; **French fries**; **Tahini**; **Taco shells**; **Potato pancakes**; **Hamburger**; **Chicken Nuggets**; **Egg rolls (veg)**; **Sugar (table, powder)**; **Syrup (table blends)**; **Mayonnaise**; **Hummus**; **Syrup (maple)**; **Sugar (brown)**; Salt (table); Barbecue sauce; Sauce (Hoisin); Sauce (fish); Soup (beef barley); Macaroni; Poppy seed; Tofu (fried); Sauces; Syrup (malt); Ketchup; Croutons; Cole slaw; Corn cakes; Soup (vegetable); Miso; Beef broth &stock; Chicken broth; Soup (chicken noodle); Soup (veg/beef); Pickle (sweet); Syrup (sorghum); Capers; Sugar (maple); Turmeric; Tabasco sauce; Chicken stock; Falafel; Mustard; Cloves; Oregano; Parsley;

Instead choose: Mints; Tomato paste; Pickle relish; Fresh Rosemary & Thyme; Soups: Clam chowder, minestrone; Sauerkraut; Herbs & Spices; Gravies; Horseradish; Soup (tomato); Sauce (tomato); Kimchi; Natto;

Alternative Therapies & Miscellaneous

Excess body weight; **2+ alcoholic drinks/day**; **Smoking/Tobacco**; **Cheese made w/whole milk**; **Deep-fried foods**; Corn syrup; Hyperthermia (avoid if extremely high blood pressure); Prescription drugs (some drugs aggravate HBP); Stress; Salted foods, nuts, etc.; Canned foods; Artificial sweeteners; Baking using butter; Birth control pills; Processed or Refined foods;

Key Nutrients & Herbal Meds

Omega-6 fatty acid (LA); **Fat (saturated)**; **Trans fatty acids**; Alcohol; Caffeine; Licorice; Sodium (salt, use spices instead or unrefined real salt/sea salt); Sugar (refined); Oxalate;

Gout (& HT)

Gout is a common and painful condition that affects your joints. It is a form of arthritis and can attack any of your joints but it often attacks joints in your big toe first.

Gout is caused by build-up of uric acid in your blood. When uric acid is stored as crystals in your joints, it creates inflammation, pain and stiffness. Uric acid builds up in your blood if you consume too much of certain foods (foods rich in purines), or if your body produces more uric acid than it eliminates. Too much alcohol consumption can adversely affect body's ability to eliminate uric acid in the blood.

You are most likely to get gout if:
- you have a family history of the disease,
- you are a man,
- you are between 40 and 50 years old,
- you drink too much alcohol,
- you are overweight,
- you consume too much of foods rich in purines (e.g., dry beans, certain fish and animal organs),
- you suffer from other medical conditions (e.g., kidney problems, high blood pressure), or
- you take certain medications (e.g., aspirin, diuretics, Niacin).

Choose these for Gout & HT

Top 5 items to choose:

Exercise; Fluids, Water & Juices; Peppers & Green Leafy Vegetables; Garlic & Onions; Fish Oil; Cranberries & Rhubarb;

Food items and actions that could improve your health (within a food group, most helpful items are listed first):

Meat, Fish & Poultry

Bluefish; Mackerel (king); Marlin; Spot; Sturgeon; Swordfish; Tilefish; Sablefish; Bass (striped); Smelt; Bass (seabass); Wolffish; Pollock; Sucker; Mullet; Bass (freshwater); Drum; White fish; Whiting; Surimi; Shad; Lobster (spiny); Milkfish; Yellowtail; Cisco; Crab (Dungeness); Salmon (pink); Trout; Tuna (blue fin); Mussels; Crab (Alaskan King); Oysters; Tilapia; Crab (snow); Dolphinfish (Mahi-Mahi); Seatrout;

Eggs, Beans, Nuts and Seeds

Seeds (chia); Egg substitute;

Fruits & Juices

Cranberries; Orange juice; Cranberry juice; Rhubarb; Cherries (especially tart, including juice); Currants (raw); Cowberries; Blackberries; Raspberries; Oranges; Grapefruit juice; Other Berries; Acerola; Lemon; Pumelo (Shaddock); Guava; Jujube (fruit); Natal Plum (Carissa); Grapefruit; Persimmons; Pineapple juice; Nectarine; Pineapple; Lime; Starfruit; Olives; Kumquats; Pomegranate; Kiwi fruit; Papaya; Pitanga; Peaches; Plum; Litchi; Abiyuch; Rowal; Apple juice; Litchi (dried); Longans; Durian; Apples; Breadfruit; Tangerines; Currants (dried); Mango; Watermelon; Apples (dried); Pears (dried); Grape juice; Pomegranate juice; Prunes (dried); Cantaloupe; Honeydew melon; *Avoid fruit juices made from concentrate or sugared*

Vegetables

Peppers (hot chili, red); Winged beans leaves; Peppers (pimento); Garlic; Taro leaves; Onions; Peppers (hot chili); Cabbage (red); Yam; Tomato juice; Balsam pear; Balsam pear leafy tips; Garden cress; Lambsquarters; Mustard spinach; Peppers (banana); Pokeberry shoots; Sesbania Flower; Taro (Tahitian); Vine spinach (Basella); Squash (Acorn); Mushrooms (Chanterelle); Cabbage (green); Amaranth leaves; Watercress; Potatoes w/skin; Cabbage (savoy); Chicory greens; Borage; Cowpeas leafy tips; Dandelion Greens; Tomatoes; Peppers (jalapeno); Celery; Bell peppers (red); Kohlrabi; Beet greens; Pumpkin flowers; Squash (Butternut); Swiss chard; Fiddlehead ferns; Parsnips; Mushrooms (shitake); Okra; Purslane; Arrowroot; Broccoli; Turnip greens; Tomatoes (sun-dried); Mushrooms (portabella); Sweet potatoes; Bell peppers (green); Endive; Kelp; Arugula; Celtuce; Green onions (scallions); Lotus root; Bok choy; Carrots; Chrysanthemum (Garland); Chrysanthemum Leaves; Cucumber with peel; Epazote; Fennel (Bulb); Hearts of palm; Various Lettuce; Nopal; Peppers (pasilla); Squash (Hubbard); Squash (Spaghetti); Sweet potatoes leaves; Wasabi root; Grape leaves; Artichoke; Brussels sprouts; Potato; Arrowhead; Beets; Taro; Broccoli (Chinese); Mushrooms (Jew's ear); Radishes; Zucchini; Cloud ear fungus; Mushrooms (Morel); Mustard greens; Eggplant; Artichoke (Jerusalem); Shallots; Kale; Turnips; Collards; Pumpkin; Rutabaga;

Breads, Grains, Cereals, Pasta

Cereal (rice crisps); Cereal (corn flakes); Bread (French/Sourdough); Cereal (shredded wheat); Cereal (cream of wheat); Buckwheat; English muffins (whole-wheat); Cereal (whole-wheat); Triticale; Rice (white); Spaghetti (whole-wheat); Toasted bread; Whole-wheat; Bread (wheat germ); Bagels; English muffins; Amaranth; Quinoa; Bread (Italian); Durum wheat; Rolls (French); Spaghetti; Wheat bran; Bulgur; Rice (wild); Rye grain; Tortillas (corn); Spelt; Sorghum grain; Bread (oat bran); Semolina; Oats; Oatmeal (cereal); Rice bran; Crackers (matzo); Wheat; Rice cakes (Brown rice);

Dairy Products, Fats & Oils

Fish oil (salmon); Fish oil (various); Cheese (Cottage); Oil (olive); Oil (flaxseed); Cream; Yogurt; Milk (1% fat); Whey (sweet); Low-fat products;

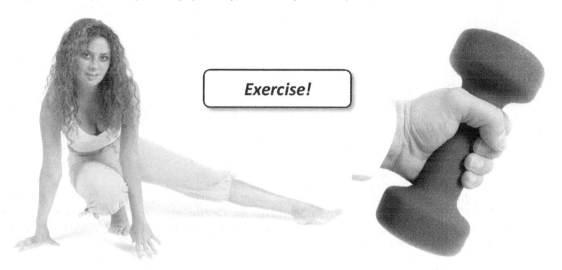

Exercise!

Desserts, Snacks, Beverages

Water; Coffee (lowers Gout risk for men, decaf in particular); Coffee (decaf); Pretzels; Tea (green);

Herbs & Spices, Fast Foods, Prepared Foods

Ginger; Parsley; Cornmeal (whole-grain); Tofu; Cayenne (red) pepper; Cinnamon; Macaroni; Corn salad; Kimchi; Croutons; Thyme (fresh);

Alternative Therapies & Miscellaneous

Exercise (i.e., cardiovascular, weight training, walking, cycling, or jogging); Wild fish and free range animals;

Key Nutrients & Herbal Meds

Omega-3 fatty acids; Celery seed; Starch/complex carbohydrates; Vitamin B-3 (Niacin in Nicotinic acid form);

Do not choose these for Gout & HT

Top 5 items to avoid:

Chocolate; Luncheon (processed) meats; Organ meats; Molasses; Sweets/Syrups; Excess body weight;

Avoid or consume much less of the following (within a food group, most harmful items are listed first):

Meat, Fish & Poultry

Bacon; Beef (cured brkfst strips); Beef jerky sticks; Beef kidneys; Beef tongue; Beerwurst beer salami; Bologna (various); Chorizo; Frankfurters; Luncheon meats; Pepperoni; Pork breakfast strips; Pork ribs; Salami; Sausages; Chicken skin; Pork liver cheese; Pastrami (turkey); Organ meats; Goose; Turkey skins; Lamb ribs; Beef chuck/brisket; Pork shoulder; Pork spare ribs; Beef (ground); Pork skins; Corned beef; Pastrami (cured beef); Pork leg/ham; Beef (cured dried); Pork; Beef ribs; Chicken wings; Chicken dark meat; Lamb; Quail; Beef shank; Squab (pigeon); Game meat; Bison/buffalo meat; Sardines; Beef; Pheasant; Duck (no skin); Croaker; Rabbit meat; Veal shoulder; Boar meat; Scallops; Goat meat; Frog legs; Venison; Fish roe; Guinea hen; Turkey dark meat; Tuna (canned); Shrimp; Beef filet mignon; Veal; Squid (Calamari); Turkey breast; White fish (smoked); Eel; Northern pike; Abalone; Perch; Carp; Whelk; Cod; Haddock; Snail; Shark; Crayfish; Veal shank; Walleye; Lobster; Chicken breast (no skin); Cuttlefish; Flatfish (flounder & sole); Conch; Crab (Blue); Orange roughy; Pout; Turbot; Pumpkinseed sunfish;

Instead choose: Pompano fish; Grouper; Snapper; Clams; Cisco (smoked); Butterfish; Scup; Tuna (yellowfin); Halibut; Octopus; Catfish; Lingcod; Burbot; Rockfish; Cusk; Anchovy; Mackerel; Herring; Caviar; Ling; Monkfish; Salmon (smoked, lox); Sheepshead;

Eggs, Beans, Nuts and Seeds

Cashew nuts; Egg yolk; Pili nuts; Brazil nuts; Coconut meat (dried); Peanuts; Seeds (sunflower); Hickory nuts; Seeds: cottonseed, pumpkin/squash, sesame, watermelon; Butternuts; Coconut meat (raw); Pine nuts; Seeds (safflower); Almonds; Beechnuts; Pecans; Pistachio nuts; Egg (hard-boiled); Walnuts (black); Egg (raw); Chickpeas; Walnuts; Hazelnuts or Filberts; Soybeans (green); Beans (baked); Lupin; Acorns; Egg (duck); Peas (split); Beans (winged); Coconut milk; Beans (lima); Pigeon peas; Lentils; other Beans; Black-eyed peas; Alfalfa sprouts; Cornnuts; Chestnuts; Peas (green); Macadamia nuts;

Instead choose: Seeds: Flaxseed, breadnut; Egg white; Peas (sugar/snap); Ginkgo nuts; Soybeans (dried); Breadfruit seeds;

Fruits & Juices

Raisins; Dates; Apricots (dried); Banana (dried); Avoid fruit Juice from concentrate or sugared;

Instead choose: Longans (dried); Peaches (dried); Plantains; Figs; Quince; Passion fruit; Avocado; Apricots; Figs (dried); Banana; Tamarind; Pears; Prune juice; Elderberries; Grapes;

Vegetables

Asparagus;

Instead choose: Leeks; Green beans; Spinach;

Breads, Grains, Cereals, Pasta

Danish pastry; **Sweet rolls**; **Donuts**; **Muffins (blueberry)**; **Muffins (oat bran)**; **Croissant**; **Granola bars**; Muffins (corn); Cereal (granola); Muffins (wheat bran); Cereal (wheat germ); Noodles (Chinese chow Mein); Bread (banana); Bread sticks; Crackers (wheat); Bread (cornbread); Noodles (egg); Biscuits; Waffles; Wheat germ; Crackers (milk); Corn; Barley; Rolls (whole-wheat dinner); Melba toast; Cereal (bran flakes); Crackers (whole-wheat);

Instead choose: Bread (white); Bread (pumpernickel); Couscous; Bread (whole-wheat); Crackers (saltines); Pasta; Spaghetti (spinach); Cereal (raisin bran); Popcorn (air popped); Oat bran; Rice (brown); Noodles (Japanese); Noodles (rice); Millet;

Dairy Products, Fats & Oils

Milk (chocolate); **Hydrogenated vegetable oil**; **Vegetable shortening**; **Margarine**; **Oils: Ucuhuba Butter, palm, Cocoa Butter, Cupu Assu**; **Fat (duck, chicken & turkey)**; **Lard**; **Cheese (American)**; **Oils: cottonseed, tea seed**; **Butter**; **Other Oils**; **Margarine-like spreads**; **Non-dairy creamers**; **Cheese (Limburger)**; **Cheese made w/whole milk**; Fat (beef/lamb/pork); Various Cheese; Cheese spread; Cream (whipped); Milk (whole); Oils: hazelnut, safflower, canola; Cheese (Ricotta); Sour cream; Milk (2% fat); Buttermilk;

Instead choose: Milk (skim);

Desserts, Snacks, Beverages

Cake (chocolate); **Chocolate mousse**; **Coffee liqueur**; **Cookies (chocolate chip)**; **Cream puffs/Éclair**; **Crème de menthe**; **Ice cream (chocolate)**; **Peanut butter**; **Puff pastry**; **Carob (candy)**; **Dessert toppings**; **Molasses**; **Candies (peanut bar)**; **Brownies**; **After-dinner mints**; **Cheesecake**; **Pies (various types)**; **Chewing gum**; **Chocolate (sweet)**; **Candies (peanut brittle)**; **Candies (sesame crunch)**; **Coffeecake**; **Halvah (candy)**; **Pie (pumpkin)**; **Chocolate (dark)**; **Pie (coconut cream)**; **Candies (caramel)**; **Frostings**; **Sherbet**; **Candies (hard)**; **Jams & Preserves**; **Jellies**; **Marshmallows**; **Cookies (butter)**; **Cakes**; **Pie (vanilla cream)**; **Pie (fried, fruit)**; **Pie (lemon meringue)**; **Pudding**; **Applesauce**; **Piña colada**; **Fruit leather/rolls**; **Ice cream (vanilla)**; **Cookies**; **Soft (carbonated) drinks**; **Ice cream cones**; **Hot chocolate**; **Pie (apple)**; **Pie (pecan)**; **Honey**; **Frozen yogurt**; **Eggnog**; **Ginger ale**; **Taro chips**; **Beer**; **80+ proof distilled alc. bev.**; **Fruit punch**; **Lemonade**; **Whiskey**; **Tonic water**; Potato sticks; Milk shakes; Pancakes; Sports drinks; Red Bull (drink); Pie crust; Tortilla chips; Popcorn (oil popped); Potato chips; Malted drinks (nonalcoholic); Wine (red); Wine (white);

Instead choose: Soy milk; Popcorn (air popped); Tea (herbal); Tea (plain);

Herbs & Spices, Fast Foods, Prepared Foods

Foie gras or liver pate; **Syrup (chocolate)**; **Hot dog**; **Teriyaki sauce**; **Salad dressings**; **Syrups**; **Tahini**; **Tofu (fried)**; **Sugar (brown)**; **Sugar (table, powder)**; **Soy sauce**; **Chicken Nuggets**; **Barbecue sauce**; **French toast**; **Cheeseburger**; Breaded shrimp; Beef & Chicken broth & stock; Sausage (meatless); Hamburger; Tempeh; Natto; Nachos; Pickle (sweet); Potato salad; Hush puppies; Onion rings; Pizza; Hummus; Mayonnaise; Soup (beef barley); Gravies (canned); Hash brown potatoes; Cottonseed meal; Soup (chicken noodle); Soup (veg/beef); Taco shells; Ketchup; Potato pancakes; Miso; Sauce (Hoisin); Fish stock; French fries; Egg rolls (veg); Corn cakes; Falafel; Sugar (maple); Poppy seed; Cocoa;

Instead <u>*choose*</u>*: Dill weed; Sage; Sauerkraut; Balsamic vinegar; Various Herbs & Spices; Horseradish; Mustard; Pickles; Sauces; Tomato paste; Vinegar; Soup (clam chowder); Cole slaw;*

Alternative Therapies & Miscellaneous

Excess body weight; **Deep Fried Food**; **2+ alcoholic drinks/day**; **Corn syrup**; **Fasting (for a specific period; do not skip meals);** Smoking/Tobacco; Aspirin; Smoked fish/foods; High dosages of Niacin; Prescription drugs (diuretics such as thiazide);

Key Nutrients & Herbal Meds

Trans fatty acids; **Alcohol**; **Brewer's Yeast**; **Fat (saturated)**; **Sugar (refined)**; Omega-6 fatty acid (LA); Purine; Sugar (fructose);

Heart Disease (& HT)

There are many forms of heart disease, but the most common form refers to narrowing of the arteries due to build-up of plaque within the arteries. This condition is thus also known as Hardening of Arteries or Atherosclerosis. As the name suggests this condition refers to a disease whereby the arteries become less flexible and hard due to buildup of fat, cholesterol and calcium on the wall of the arteries. Overtime the arteries can get narrower (or blocked) leading to less (or no) oxygen flow to various parts of our body.

In case of arteries that supply blood to heart, this condition is known as Coronary Heart Disease (or coronary artery disease), and can lead to chest pain, heart failure (also known as congestive heart failure) and heart attack. In case of arteries that supply blood to the brain, it can lead to a stroke.

If the buildup on the walls of the arteries breaks off from the arteries it can lead to a blood clot which can completely block flow of blood (oxygen) to a specific part of our body. Unfortunately, for most people this condition is unknown until there is a medical emergency. Hardening of the coronary arteries is the leading cause of death for both men and women in the US.

While the cause of atherosclerosis is unknown, it is believed that it starts with damage to the interior walls of the arteries. Factors that could lead to this damage include smoking, high cholesterol and other fats in the blood, high blood pressure, and high blood sugar level.

In addition to the above factors, there are a number of other known risk factors including: obesity, lack of exercise, poor diet, increasing age (over 45 for men, 55 for women), family history of the disease at an early age, high triglycerides level (especially for women), excess alcohol consumption, stress and sleep apnea.

Atherosclerosis is a common health problem, but can be prevented or delayed through diet and life style changes, and addressing the risk factors.

Choose these for Heart Disease & HT

Top 5 items to consume:

Fish & Shellfish; Fish Oil; Garlic; Mushrooms & Peppers; Soybeans; & Exercise;

Food items and actions that could improve your health (within a food group, most helpful items are listed first):

Meat, Fish & Poultry (2+ fish meals per week; up to 6 oz. of meat/poultry/fish per day)

Anchovy; Bluefish; Cisco (smoked); Mackerel; Mackerel (king); Marlin; Salmon (pink); Spot; Sturgeon; Swordfish; Trout; Tuna (blue fin); White fish; Herring; Sablefish; Tilefish; Salmon (smoked, Lox); Mussels; Caviar; Bass (striped); Smelt; Tuna (yellowfin); Halibut; Bass (seabass); Wolffish; Pollock; Sucker; Mullet; Bass (freshwater); Drum; Oysters; Whiting; Crab (Dungeness); Lobster (spiny); Shad; Milkfish; Yellowtail; Cisco; Crab (Alaskan King); Surimi; Pompano fish; Tilapia; Seatrout; Walleye; Dolphinfish (Mahi-Mahi); White fish (smoked); Grouper; Snapper; Flatfish (flounder & sole); Butterfish; Scup; Catfish; Lingcod; Burbot; Rockfish; Crab (snow); Cusk; Carp; Perch; Haddock; Octopus; Northern pike; Cod; Ling; Monkfish; Sheepshead; Pumpkinseed sunfish; Clams; Conch; Pout; Turbot; Tuna (canned); Snail; Orange roughy; Shark; Fish roe; Sardines; Chicken breast (no skin); Beef filet mignon; Crab (Blue); Scallops; Lobster; Pheasant breast; Quail breast; Crayfish; Whelk; Veal loin; Veal shank; Cuttlefish; Beef rib eye; Eel; Caribou meat; Turkey breast;

Eggs, Beans, Nuts and Seeds

Soybeans (dried); Peas (sugar/snap); Seeds (chia); Peas (green); Beans: lima, yardlong; Lentils; Peas (split); Various Beans; Black-eyed peas; Pigeon peas; Lupin; Seeds (flaxseed); Chickpeas; Egg substitute; Soybeans (green); Egg white; Seeds (breadnut tree);

Fruits & Juices (5+ servings per day)

Blackberries; Cowberries; Apricots; Cantaloupe; Currants (raw); Guava; Peaches; Plum; Watermelon; Passion fruit; Strawberries; Boysenberries; Papaya; Pitanga; Pomegranate; Persimmons; Raspberries (black in particular); Berries; Rhubarb; Durian; Acerola; Plantains; Lemon; Lime; Natal Plum (Carissa); Starfruit; Mango; Apples; Cranberry juice; Pears; Olives; Pumelo (Shaddock); Currants (dried); Jujube (fruit); Orange juice; Nectarine; Banana; Oranges; Kumquats; Abiyuch; Apple juice; Grapefruit juice; Grapes; Cherries; Rowal; Raisins; Honeydew melon; Pineapple; Pineapple juice; Tangerines; Breadfruit; Dried Fruits; Grapefruit (pink in particular); Pomegranate juice; Kiwi fruit; Quince; Avocado; Prune juice; **Avoid sugared or made from concentrate juices;**

Vegetables

Garlic (4 grams of minced fresh garlic or 8 milligrams of essential oil daily); **Winged beans leaves**; **Mushrooms: portabella, shitake, Chanterelle**; **Peppers (pimento)**; **Peppers (jalapeno)**; **Arrowroot**; **Chicory greens**; **Taro leaves**; **Tomatoes (sun-dried)**; **Peppers (hot chili, red)**; **Cloud ear fungus**; **Endive**; **Artichoke**; **Onions**; Amaranth leaves; Arugula; Asparagus; Balsam pear leafy tips; Beet greens; Bell peppers (red); Bok choy; Broccoli (Chinese); Various Cabbage; Chrysanthemum (Garland); Chrysanthemum Leaves; Collards; Dandelion Greens; Epazote; Garden cress; Kale; Lambsquarters; Various Lettuce; Mustard greens; Mustard spinach; Various Peppers; Pokeberry shoots; Pumpkin; Various Squash; Sweet potatoes leaves; Taro (Tahitian); Tomato juice; Tomatoes; Turnip greens; Vine spinach (Basella); Watercress; Green onions (scallions); Grape leaves; Borage; Swiss chard; Celtuce; Kelp; Sweet potatoes; Mushrooms (Morel); Cowpeas leafy tips; Pumpkin flowers; Leeks; Purslane; Zucchini; Other vegetables;

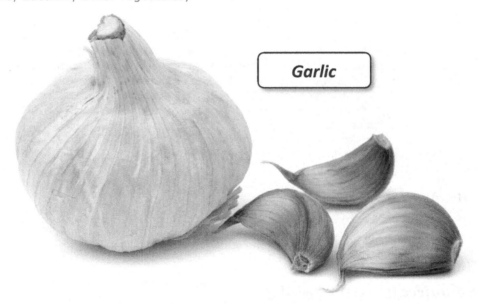

Garlic

Breads, Grains, Cereals, Pasta (Six servings of whole grains per day)

Oats; Triticale; Rice cakes (Brown rice); Buckwheat; English muffins (whole-wheat); Oat bran; Couscous; Sorghum grain; Durum wheat; Barley; Rice (brown); Rye grain; Quinoa; Oatmeal (cereal); Rice bran; Wheat bran; Whole-wheat; Millet; Spaghetti (spinach); Rice (wild); Spaghetti (whole-wheat); Bread (wheat germ); Bread (whole-wheat); Cereal (corn flakes); Corn bran; Spelt; Bulgur; Corn;

Dairy Products, Fats & Oils

Fish oil (salmon); **Fish oil (cod liver)**; **Other Fish oil**; **Oil (olive)**; Oil (flaxseed); Cheese (Cottage); Cream; Yogurt; Fat-free or low fat products;

Desserts, Snacks, Beverages

Tea (green); Wine (red); Tea (plain); Water;

Herbs & Spices, Fast Foods, Prepared Foods

Parsley; Soups: minestrone, clam chowder; Cayenne (red) pepper; Cinnamon; Ginger; Tomato paste; Fish stock; Coriander/Cilantro; Tofu; Soup (vegetable); Corn salad; Soup (veg/beef); Basil (fresh); Soup (tomato); Thyme (fresh); Cocoa; Saffron; Turmeric; Cottonseed meal; Tempeh; Dill weed; Miso; Succotash; Rosemary (fresh); Mints; Spearmint (fresh); Peppermint;

Alternative Therapies & Miscellaneous

Exercise (including cardiovascular, weight training, walk, wheel, or jog); **Wild fish and free range animals**; Organically grown foods; Mediterranean diet; Ornish Plan & Diet; Tai Chi; Yoga; Fat-free or low fat products;

Key Nutrients & Herbal Meds

Omega-3 fatty acids; Hawthorn (In berries form or tea from dried leaves and flowers, do not take with other heart medications); Vitamin B-3 (Niacin, in nicotinic acid form, not recommended as supplement or drug); Astragalus (Herb); DHEA (dehydroepiandosterone); Flavonoids; Ginseng (Siberian); Guggul; Lycopene; Goji berry;

Do not choose these for Heart Disease & HT

Top 5 items to avoid:

Sweets; Luncheon/Processed Meats; Fast Foods; Butternuts, Pili Nuts & Hickory Nuts; Cheese; & Excess Weight;

Avoid or consume much less of the following (within a food group, most harmful items are listed first):

Meat, Fish & Poultry

Beef jerky sticks; Beef tongue; Salami; Bologna; Chicken heart; Chorizo; Frankfurters; Lamb tongue; Luncheon meats; Organ Meats; Pepperoni; Pork breakfast strips; Pork headcheese; Pork ribs; Pork skins; Sausages; Pastrami; Goose; Bacon; Chicken skin; Pork spare ribs; Turkey skins; Corned beef; Chicken wings; Lamb ribs; Chicken dark meat; Beef chuck/brisket; Pork shoulder; Cured meats; Beef ribs; Beef (ground); Lamb loin; Squab (pigeon); Lamb (ground); Pork back ribs; Lamb shoulder; Pork; Quail; Beef; Game Meat; Abalone; Duck (no skin); Bison/buffalo meat; Frog legs; Rabbit meat; Venison;

*Instead **Choose**: Veal shoulder; Beef round steak; Turkey dark meat; Shrimp; Beef top sirloin; Pheasant; Goat meat; Squid (Calamari); Croaker; Guinea hen; Lamb leg;*

Eggs, Beans, Nuts and Seeds

Butternuts; Pili nuts; Hickory nuts; Seeds (watermelon); Egg (hard-boiled); Pine nuts; Egg (raw); Coconut meat (dried); Coconut meat (raw); Beechnuts; Egg yolk; Seeds: cottonseed, safflower; Pistachio nuts; Egg (duck); Peanuts; Cashew nuts; Walnuts (black); Brazil nuts; Acorns; Walnuts; Coconut milk; Seeds (sunflower); Hazelnuts or Filberts; Cornnuts; Chestnuts; Soy milk; Seeds: pumpkin/squash, sesame; Alfalfa sprouts; Almonds; Pecans; Breadfruit seeds;

*Instead **Choose**: Ginkgo nuts; Macadamia nuts;*

Fruits & Juices

Avoid sugared or made from concentrate juices;

*Instead **Choose**: Litchi (dried); Dates; Tamarind; Figs (dried); Figs;*

Breads, Grains, Cereals, Pasta

Bread (banana); Cereal (granola); Croissant; Danish pastry; Sweet rolls; Waffles; Crackers (wheat); Biscuits; Bread (cornbread); Donuts; Granola bars; Various Muffins; Crackers (milk); Crackers (whole-wheat); Bread sticks; Crackers (saltines); Rolls (Kaiser); Noodles (Chinese chow Mein); Noodles (egg); Bread (white); Rolls (whole-wheat dinner); Rolls (hamburger/hot dog); Melba toast; Tortillas (corn); Bagels; English muffins; Cereal (cream of wheat); Rolls (French); Breads: Italian, pumpernickel, oat bran; Cereal (rice crisps); Pasta; Crackers (matzo); Cereal (shredded wheat); Cereal (wheat germ); Cereal (bran flakes); Wheat; Toasted bread; Cereal (raisin bran); Noodles (rice);

*Instead **Choose**: Cereal (whole-wheat); Cornmeal (whole-grain); Rice (white); Semolina; Spaghetti; Amaranth; Wheat germ; Bread (French/Sourdough); Noodles (Japanese);*

Dairy Products, Fats & Oils

Cheese (American); Cheese (Cream); Cream (whipped); Fat (chicken, duck, turkey); Margarine-like spreads; Oils: corn, poppy seed, sesame, tea seed, tomato seeds); Cheese: Roquefort, Pimento; Other Oils; Cheese: Romano, Brie, Cheddar, Goat); Cheese spread; Other Cheese; Fat (beef/lamb/pork); Butter; Hydrogenated vegetable oil; Lard; Margarine; Non-dairy creamers; Vegetable shortening; Milk (whole); Milk (chocolate); Sour cream; Milk (skim); Milk (1% fat); Milk (2% fat); Buttermilk;

Instead <u>*Choose*</u>*: Oil (canola); Whey (sweet);*

Desserts, Snacks, Beverages

Sherbet; After-dinner mints; Brownies; Cakes; Candies; Cheesecake; Chewing gum; Chocolate mousse; Coffee liqueur; Coffeecake; Cookies; Cream puffs/Éclair; Crème de menthe; Dessert toppings; Frostings; Fruit leather/rolls; Halvah (candy); Honey; Ice creams; Ice cream cones; Jams & Preserves; Jellies; Marshmallows; Peanut butter; Pies; Pie crust; Potato sticks; Puff pastry; Taro chips; Pudding; Chocolate (sweet); Tortilla chips; Frozen yogurt; Popcorn (oil popped); Pancakes; Eggnog; Chocolate (dark); Potato chips; Piña colada; Applesauce; Soft (carbonated) drinks; Fruit punch; Hot chocolate; Lemonade; Ginger ale; Molasses; Milk shakes; Tonic water; Pretzels; Sports drinks; Malted drinks (nonalcoholic); Popcorn (air popped); 80+ proof distilled alc. bev.; Whiskey; Wine (white); Beer;

Instead <u>*Choose*</u>*: Coffee (decaf); Red Bull (drink); Coffee; Grape juice; Tea (herbal);*

Herbs & Spices, Fast Foods, Prepared Foods

Breaded shrimp; Cheeseburger; Foie gras or liver pate; French toast; Hash brown potatoes; Hush puppies; Nachos; Onion rings; Pizza; Potato pancakes; Potato salad; Salad dressings; Syrup (chocolate); Taco shells; Syrup (maple); Hot dog; Hamburger; Syrup (table blends); French fries; Sausage (meatless); Teriyaki sauce; Sugar (table, powder); Mayonnaise; Chicken Nuggets; Sugar (brown); Syrup (sorghum); Soy sauce; Hummus; Natto; Barbecue sauce; Salt (table); Syrup (malt); Egg rolls (veg); Sauce (Hoisin); Pickle (sweet); Gravies (canned); Poppy seed; Corn cakes; Sauce (fish); Tahini; Sugar (maple); Chicken broth; Soup (chicken noodle); Ketchup; Sauces; Tofu (fried); Chicken stock; Macaroni; Cole slaw; Tabasco sauce; Croutons; Sauerkraut;

Instead <u>*Choose*</u>*: Pepper (black); Sauce (tomato); Sage; Pickle; Balsamic Vinegar; Herbs & Spices; Horseradish; Vinegar; Mustard; Kimchi; Falafel; Soup (beef barley); Capers;*

Alternative Therapies & Miscellaneous

Excess body weight; Corn syrup; Smoking/Tobacco; Deep-fried foods; Baking using butter; Canned foods; 2+ alcoholic drinks/day; Cheese made w/whole milk; Artificial sweeteners; Stress;

Key Nutrients & Herbal Meds

Trans fatty acids; Omega-6 fatty acid (LA); Fat (saturated, Limit to less than 7% of daily calorie); Cholesterol (Limit to less than 200mg per day); Sugar (refined); Pine oil (damage is possible when taken internally); Sugar (total); Alcohol;

Diabetes Type 2 (& HT)

Diabetes is a disorder that refers to our body's inability to use or convert food to the fuel needed by our cells.

Insulin is a hormone that helps the glucose (sugar) get into the body cells. In diabetes, the body is unable to create or properly use insulin. Without insulin, glucose stays in the blood and eventually makes its way to the urine, instead of serving as fuel to our muscles, tissues and brain.

There are different types of diabetes but the most common one is Diabetes Type 2 which represents 90-95% of diabetes cases, and is the focus of this section.

You are at most risk to develop diabetes Type 2 if you are obese. Your risk increases as you get older, if you are a member of a US minority group, are physically inactive, have a family history of the disease, have high blood pressure, have low level of good cholesterol, or have a high level of triglycerides.

Over time, excessive blood sugar level can cause serious health problems, in particular heart related issues. Over 65% of those with diabetes die from heart disease or stroke.

While there is no cure for diabetes type 2, there are numerous tools such as nutrition and exercise to help with the management of this disorder. In addition to managing the blood sugar level, the goal of diabetes management includes control of blood pressure, and cholesterol levels.

Choose these for Diabetes (Type 2) & HT

Top 5 items to consume:

> Fish; Cod liver fish oil; Shellfish; Soybeans; Mushrooms; & Exercise;

Food items and actions that could improve your health (within a food group, most helpful items are listed first):

Meat, Fish & Poultry

Anchovy; Bluefish; Cisco (smoked); Mackerel; Mackerel (king); Marlin; Salmon (pink); Spot; Sturgeon; Swordfish; Trout; Tuna (blue fin); White fish; Herring; Sablefish; Tilefish; Salmon (smoked, Lox); Tuna (yellowfin); Halibut; Bass (seabass); Wolffish; Smelt; Drum; Sucker; Oysters; Mullet; Bass (striped); Pollock; Whiting; Shad; Bass (freshwater); Cisco; Mussels; Crab (Alaskan King); Surimi; Lobster (spiny); Milkfish; Pompano fish; Tilapia; White fish (smoked); Snapper; Catfish; Chicken breast (no skin); Yellowtail; Flatfish (flounder & sole); Carp; Grouper; Crab (Dungeness); Seatrout; Cusk; Dolphinfish (Mahi-Mahi); Walleye; Rockfish; Burbot; Scup; Lingcod; Perch; Tuna (canned); Butterfish; Crab (snow); Ling; Beef filet mignon; Northern pike; Octopus; Clams; Sardines; Cod; Haddock; Shark; Caviar; Monkfish; Pumpkinseed sunfish; Sheepshead; Pout; Beef; Conch; Eel; Orange roughy; Turbot; Veal shank; Snail; Quail breast; Pheasant breast; Veal loin; Liver; Caribou meat; Crab (Blue); Lobster; Veal shoulder; Scallops; Whelk; Goat meat; Cuttlefish; Fish roe; Bear meat; Pheasant; Turkey dark meat; Turkey breast; Pork loin/sirloin; Lamb leg; Croaker; Venison; Guinea hen;

Eggs, Beans, Nuts and Seeds

Soybeans (dried); Seeds: chia, flaxseed; Peas: sugar/snap, green, split; Various Beans; Black-eyed peas; Soybeans (green); Alfalfa sprouts; Pigeon peas; Chickpeas; Egg white; Lupin; Macadamia nuts; Lentils; Hazelnuts or Filberts; Seeds (breadnut tree); Egg substitute; Seeds (sunflower); Ginkgo nuts;

Fruits & Juices

Pitanga; Apricots; Cantaloupe; Elderberries; Grapefruit; Guava; Acerola; Passion fruit; Persimmons; Mango; Berries; Lemon; Apricots (dried); Durian; Kumquats; Papaya; Lime; Starfruit; Pumelo (Shaddock); Plantains; Jujube (fruit); Abiyuch; Natal Plum (Carissa); Olives; Rhubarb; Rowal; Peaches; Nectarine; Plum; Apples; Currants (raw); Watermelon; Tangerines; Peaches (dried); Kiwi fruit; Pears; Avocado; Oranges; Orange juice; Banana; Grapefruit juice; Prunes (dried); Apple juice; Honeydew melon; Pineapple juice; Pineapple; Banana (dried); Pomegranate; Grape juice; Cranberry juice; Pomegranate juice; Apples (dried); Cherries; Quince; Longans (dried); _**Avoid fruit juices made from concentrate or with added sugar**_

Vegetables

Various Mushrooms; **Winged beans leaves**; **Peppers (jalapeno)**; **Peppers (pimento)**; **Chicory greens**; **Taro leaves**; **Peppers (hot chili)**; **Broccoli**; **Cauliflower**; **Endive**; **Garlic**; Amaranth leaves; Arugula; Asparagus; Balsam pear leafy tips; Beet greens; Bell peppers; Bok choy; Borage; Broccoli (Chinese); Brussels sprouts; Cabbage; Carrots; Celtuce; Chrysanthemum (Garland); Chrysanthemum Leaves; Collards; Dandelion Greens; Garden cress; Green beans; Green onions (scallions); Kale; Lambsquarters; Leeks; Various Lettuce; Mustard greens; Mustard spinach; Okra; Peppers; Pokeberry shoots; Pumpkin flowers; Purslane; Spinach; Various Squash; Sweet potatoes leaves; Swiss chard; Taro (Tahitian); Tomatoes; Turnip greens; Vine spinach (Basella); Watercress; Zucchini; Parsnips; Potato; Grape leaves; Kohlrabi; Mushrooms (Jew's ear); Epazote; Sweet potatoes; Cowpeas leafy tips; Kelp; Yam; Tomato juice; Radishes; Other Vegetables;

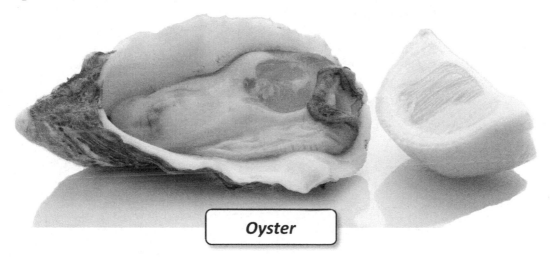

Oyster

Breads, Grains, Cereals, Pasta

Rice bran; Buckwheat; English muffins (whole-wheat); Bread (wheat germ); Cereal (corn flakes); Corn bran; Rice cakes (Brown rice); Rice (wild); Rye grain; Cereals: shredded wheat, rice crisps, whole-wheat; Spaghetti (whole-wheat); Spelt; Whole-wheat; Oatmeal (cereal); Triticale; Durum wheat; Cereal (raisin bran); Oats; Bulgur; Quinoa; Bread (pumpernickel); Sorghum grain; Toasted bread; Tortillas (corn); Bread (French/Sourdough); Wheat; Wheat germ; Corn; Noodles (Chinese chow Mein); Pasta; Barley; Spaghetti (spinach); Spaghetti; Rice (brown);

Dairy Products, Fats & Oils

Fish oil (cod liver); **Fish oil (salmon)**; **Oil (flaxseed)**; **Fish oil (sardine)**; Other Fish oil; Oil (olive); Cheese (Cottage);

Desserts, Snacks, Beverages

Coffee; Coffee (decaf); Tea (green); Water;

Herbs & Spices, Fast Foods, Prepared Foods

Cinnamon; Parsley; Soups: minestrone, vegetable; Coriander/Cilantro; Thyme (fresh); Cayenne (red) pepper; Soup (veg/beef); Corn salad; Basil (fresh); Ginger; Dill weed; Cornmeal (whole-grain); Rosemary (fresh); Spearmint (fresh); Tofu; Falafel; Fish stock; Soup (clam chowder); Cottonseed meal; Peppermint; Sage; Succotash; Kimchi; Soup (beef barley); Cocoa; Mints; Tomato paste; Croutons; Tempeh; Pepper (black); Egg rolls (veg);

Alternative Therapies & Miscellaneous

Consult your doctor (maintain annual physical exam; get vaccinated; monitor eyes, foot, blood pressure ...); Exercise (including cardiovascular, weight training, walk, wheel, or jog); Wild fish and free range animals; Eat smaller more frequent meals; Glucomannan; Organically grown foods; Exposure to sun;

Key Nutrients & Herbal Meds

Omega-3 fatty acids; Brewer's Yeast; Vitamin B-3 (Niacin, in nicotinic acid form, not recommended as supplement or drug); Chromium; Fat (monounsaturated); Fat (polyunsaturated); Fiber; Ginseng (Siberian); Goji berry; Gymnema; Psyllium; Vitamin A; Zinc; Beta Carotene;

Do not choose these for Diabetes (Type 2) & HT

Top 5 items to avoid:

Hydrogenated Vegetable Oil; Chocolate; Sweets; Processed Luncheon Meats; Animal Fat; & Excess weight;

Avoid or consume much less of the following (within a food group, most harmful items are listed first):

Meat, Fish & Poultry

Chicken & Turkey skins; Salami; Bologna; Frankfurters; Luncheon meats; Pepperoni; Sausages; Pastrami; Chorizo; Beef jerky sticks; Beef tongue; Pork skins; Bacon; Lamb brain; Veal thymus; Pork breakfast strips; Beef kidneys; Veal lungs; Organ Meats; Corned beef; Cured Meats; Lamb ribs; Pork ribs/spare ribs; Goose; Lamb loin; Pork; Lamb; Beaver meat; Beef chuck/brisket; Frog legs; Squid (Calamari);

Instead Choose: Beef shank; Boar meat; Shrimp; Quail; Bison/buffalo meat; Abalone; Crayfish; Rabbit meat; Chicken dark meat; Duck (no skin); Squab (pigeon); Beef ribs; Beef (ground); Chicken wings;

Eggs, Beans, Nuts and Seeds

Coconut meat (dried); Coconut meat (raw); Pili nuts; Egg (raw); Egg (hard-boiled); Seeds (cottonseed); Coconut milk; Brazil nuts; Butternuts; Beechnuts; Seeds (pumpkin/squash); Cashew nuts; Hickory nuts; Seeds: watermelon, safflower, sesame; Egg yolk; Egg (duck); Pistachio nuts; Acorns; Pine nuts; Walnuts (black); Peanuts; Soy milk; Chestnuts;

Instead Choose: Almonds; Walnuts; Pecans; Cornnuts; Breadfruit seeds;

Fruits & Juices

Avoid sugared or made from concentrate juices;

Instead Choose: Figs; Breadfruit; Litchi; Litchi (dried); Prune juice; Longans; Grapes;

Breads, Grains, Cereals, Pasta

Croissant; Danish pastry; Donuts; Muffins (blueberry); Sweet rolls; Bread (cornbread); Crackers (wheat); Waffles; Cereal (bran flakes); Muffins (corn); Granola bars; Muffins (wheat bran); Muffins (oat bran); Crackers (milk); Bread (white); Rolls (Kaiser); Biscuits; Bread (banana); Cereal (granola); Crackers (saltines); Rolls (hamburger/hot dog); Rice (white); Crackers (whole-wheat); Melba toast; Noodles (egg); Bread sticks; Crackers (matzo); Wheat bran;

Instead Choose: Cereal (cream of wheat); Bread (whole-wheat, whole-grain in particular); Oat bran; Millet; Bread (Italian); English muffins; Semolina; Bagels; Popcorn (oil popped); Cereal (wheat germ); Noodles (Japanese); Couscous; Amaranth; Bread (oat bran); Rolls (whole-wheat dinner); Noodles (rice);

Dairy Products, Fats & Oils

Hydrogenated vegetable oil; **Fat (chicken, duck, turkey)**; **Lard**; **Non-dairy creamers**; **Oil (Ucuhuba Butter)**; **Vegetable shortening**; **Cream (whipped)**; **Margarine**; **Oil (coconut)**; **Fat (beef/lamb/pork)**; **Oil (Cocoa Butter)**; **Oil (Babassu)**; **Butter**; **Oils: Cupu Assu, palm, Shea nut, Tea seed, Cottonseed**; **Milk (chocolate)**; **Cheese (American)**; **Margarine-like spreads**; **Cheese: Feta, Romano, Cream**; **Cheese spread**; Other Cheese; Other Oils; Sour cream; Milk (whole); Milk (skim); Whey (sweet); Oil (almonds); Milk (1% fat); Milk (2% fat);

*Instead **Choose**: Oils: canola, safflower, wheat germ, hazelnut; Buttermilk; Cream; Yogurt;*

Desserts, Snacks, Beverages

Sherbet; **After-dinner mints**; **Brownies**; **Cakes**; **Candies**; **Cheesecake**; **Chewing gum**; **Chocolate mousse**; **Coffee liqueur**; **Cookies**; **Cream puffs/Éclair**; **Crème de menthe**; **Dessert toppings**; **Frostings**; **Fruit leather/rolls**; **Honey**; **Ice creams**; **Ice cream cones**; **Jams & Preserves**; **Jellies**; **Marshmallows**; **Pies**; **Puff pastry**; **Frozen yogurt**; **Coffeecake**; **Pudding**; **Molasses**; **Chocolate (sweet)**; **Candies (peanut bar)**; **Piña colada**; **Milk shakes**; **Chocolate (dark)**; **Halvah (candy)**; **Pancakes**; **Eggnog**; **Applesauce**; **Soft (carbonated) drinks**; **Ginger ale**; **Hot chocolate**; **Tonic water**; **Fruit punch**; **Lemonade**; **Sports drinks**; Red Bull (drink); Potato sticks; Pie crust; 80+ proof distilled alc. bev.; Whiskey; Candies (sesame crunch); Taro chips; Malted drinks (nonalcoholic); Pretzels; Wine (red); Wine (white); Peanut butter; Beer; Tea (plain);

*Instead **Choose**: Popcorn (air popped); Potato chips; Popcorn (oil popped); Tahini; Tortilla chips; Tea (herbal);*

Herbs & Spices, Fast Foods, Prepared Foods

Salad dressings; **Syrups**; **Pizza**; **Hot dog**; **Teriyaki sauce**; **Nachos**; **Sugar (brown)**; **Sugar (table, powder)**; **Cheeseburger**; **Breaded shrimp**; **French toast**; **Barbecue sauce**; **Potato salad**; **Hush puppies**; **Sauce (Hoisin)**; **Soy sauce**; **Hamburger**; **Pickle (sweet)**; Ketchup; Chicken Nuggets; Mayonnaise; Onion rings; Potato pancakes; Sugar (maple); Taco shells; Foie gras or liver pate; Hummus; Sausage (meatless); Hash brown potatoes; French fries; Sauce (cheese); Sauces; Corn cakes; Poppy seed; Chicken broth & stock; Soup (chicken noodle); Natto; Macaroni; Beef broth & stock; Tofu (fried);

*Instead **Choose**: Sauerkraut; Balsamic vinegar; Capers; Herbs & Spices; Gravies; Horseradish; Mustard; Pickle; Salt; Vinegar; Miso; Cole slaw;*

Alternative Therapies & Miscellaneous

Excess body weight; **Corn syrup**; **Smoking/Tobacco**; **Deep-fried foods**; **2+ alcoholic drinks/day**; **Artificial sweeteners**; **Baking using butter**; **Cheese made w/whole milk**; **Fasting (for a specific period)**; Saccharine (NutraSweet); Aspartame (Equal); Fat-free or low fat products; Abrupt changes in diet/exercise; Stress; Processed or Refined foods;

Key Nutrients & Herbal Meds

Fat (saturated); **Trans fatty acids**; **Sugar (refined)**; **Omega-6 fatty acid (LA)**; **Cholesterol**; **Sugar (total)**; Alcohol;

Obesity or Excess Body Weight (& HT)

Obesity is defined as having too much body fat. It normally occurs when you continue to eat more calories than your body burns through exercise and normal daily activities. The unused calories are then stored as fat in your body leading to obesity.

Obesity is a risk factor for many diseases and illnesses including certain types of cancer. However, even a modest reduction in body fat (5 to 10% weight loss) can reduce your risk or delay illnesses caused by obesity.

The common way to measure obesity is body mass index (BMI). BMI is calculated by multiplying your weight in pounds by 703, divided by the square of your height in inches. For example a 6 feet tall man who weighs 190 pounds, has a BMI of 25.8. In the metric system, BMI is your weight in kilograms divided by the square of your height in meters.

Your BMI is considered normal if it is between 18.5 and 24.9. You are obese if your BMI is 30 or higher. You have excess body weight if your BMI is between 24.9 and 30.

Risk factors that can lead to obesity include: lack of physical exercise, overeating (e.g., oversized portions, recovery from quitting smoking), poor diet (e.g., eating high-fat foods), genetic or family history, pregnancy (inability to lose weight after giving birth), hormone problems, certain medications and illnesses, emotional issues (boredom, anger or stress), growing older, and lack of sleep.

Choose these for   Excess body weight & HT

Top 5 items to consume:

Fish; Shellfish; Fish Oil; Garlic, Artichoke & Mushrooms; Wild fish and free range animals; & Exercise;

Food items and actions that could improve your health (within a food group, most helpful items are listed first):

**Meat, Fish & Poultry** (5.5 oz. of meat/fowl/fish or beans per day)

Bluefish; Mackerel (king); Marlin; Salmon (pink); Spot; Sturgeon; Swordfish; Trout; Tuna (blue fin); White fish; Herring; Tilefish; Mackerel; Sablefish; Cisco (smoked); Bass (striped); Smelt; Tuna (yellowfin); Anchovy; Halibut; Bass (seabass); Wolffish; Pollock; Sucker; Bass (freshwater); Drum; Whiting; Cisco; Mullet; Surimi; Seatrout; Milkfish; Walleye; Snapper; Yellowtail; Tilapia; Grouper; Caviar; Mussels; Shad; Lingcod; Salmon (smoked, Lox); Pompano fish; Burbot; Dolphinfish (Mahi-Mahi); Rockfish; Oysters; Flatfish (flounder & sole); Catfish; Scup; Cusk; Perch; Butterfish; Northern pike; Carp; Cod; Lobster (spiny); Sheepshead; Ling; Crab (Dungeness); Haddock; Monkfish; Chicken breast (no skin); Pumpkinseed sunfish; Pout; Orange roughy; Turbot; Crab (snow); White fish (smoked); Crab (Alaskan King); Octopus; Tuna (canned); Fish roe; Clams; Pheasant breast; Shark; Quail breast; Conch; Turkey breast; Lobster; Snail; Scallops; Sardines; Crab (Blue);

**Eggs, Beans, Nuts and Seeds** (5.5 oz. of meat/fowl/fish or beans per day)

Beans: navy, yellow; Lentils; Peas: split, green; Beans: yardlong. pinto; Peas (sugar/snap); Various Beans; Alfalfa sprouts; Seeds (chia); Black-eyed peas; Pigeon peas; Soybeans (dried); Seeds (flaxseed); Lupin; Egg substitute;

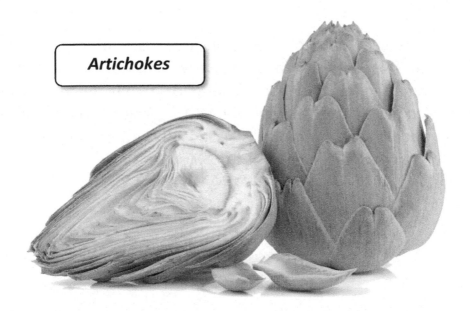

Artichokes

Choose This not That for **High Triglycerides**   Page 72

Fruits & Juices (2 cups of fruits & juices per day)

Blackberries; Raspberries; Passion fruit; Lemon; Guava; Berries; Lime; Starfruit; Acerola; Pitanga; Pumelo (Shaddock); Natal Plum (Carissa); Currants (raw); Kiwi fruit; Olives; Rhubarb; Durian; Abiyuch; Kumquats; Cantaloupe; Papaya; Apricots; Apples; Oranges; Grapefruit; Jujube (fruit); Pineapple; Watermelon; Nectarine; Peaches; Plum; Banana; Persimmons; Honeydew melon; Rowal; Pears; Mango; Tangerines; Breadfruit; Prunes (dried); Banana (dried); Pomegranate; Apricots (dried); Peaches (dried); **Avoid sugared or made from concentrate juices;**

Vegetables (2.5 cups per day)

Garlic; **Artichoke**; **Cloud ear fungus**; **Mushrooms (shitake)**; Mushrooms (Chanterelle); Peppers (pasilla); Potato; Winged beans leaves; Bell peppers (green); Grape leaves; Broccoli; Taro leaves; Peppers (pimento); Mushrooms (portabella); Peppers; Onions; Squash (Acorn); Chicory greens; Parsnips; Sweet potatoes leaves; Carrots; Balsam pear leafy tips; Lambsquarters; Mustard greens; Mustard spinach; Turnip greens; Cabbage (savoy); Squash (Butternut); Collards; Dandelion Greens; Mushrooms (Morel); Endive; Spinach; Cabbage (green); Brussels sprouts; Broccoli (Chinese); Kohlrabi; Celery; Cucumber with peel; Yam; Chrysanthemum (Garland); Chrysanthemum Leaves; Squash (Hubbard); Balsam pear; Green beans; Cabbage (red); Okra; Mushrooms (Jew's ear); Fiddlehead ferns; Green onions (scallions); Bell peppers (red); Garden cress; Kale; Vine spinach (Basella); Amaranth leaves; Bok choy; Arrowroot; Tomatoes (sun-dried); Cauliflower; Beet greens; Pokeberry shoots; Taro (Tahitian); Epazote; other vegetables;

Breads, Grains, Cereals, Pasta (6 oz. of grains/day; 3+ oz. from whole grains)

Corn bran; Buckwheat; Triticale; Rice (brown);

Dairy Products, Fats & Oils (3 cups of low fat products per day)

Fish oil (salmon); **Fish oil (cod liver)**; **Other fish oil**; Oil (flaxseed); Yogurt;

Desserts, Snacks, Beverages

Tea (green); Water;

Herbs & Spices, Fast Foods, Prepared Foods

Cayenne (red) pepper; **Cinnamon**; Ginger; Soup (clam chowder); Soup (minestrone); Fish stock; Soup (vegetable); Soup (tomato); Thyme (fresh);

Alternative Therapies & Miscellaneous

Exercise (include sit-ups and lower back exercises); **Exercise - cardiovascular**; **Exercise - weight training**; **Walk, wheel, or jog (Try to reach 10,000 steps per day gradually. Suck stomach in while running)**; **Wild fish and free range animals**; Choose smaller food portions (choose smaller meals, eat slowly); Eat breakfast; Weigh yourself daily; Organic cold-pressed oils;

Key Nutrients & Herbal Meds

Omega-3 fatty acids; Vitamin B-3 (Niacin; in nicotinic acid form, not recommended as supplement or drug); Fiber; Psyllium;

Do not choose these for   Excess body weight & HT

Top 5 items to avoid:

Fast Foods; Sweets; Butter, Margarine & Cheese;
Luncheon (Processed) Meats; Hydrogenated
vegetable oil;

Avoid or consume much less of the following (within a food group, most harmful items are listed first):

Meat, Fish & Poultry

Bacon; Beef jerky sticks; Beef tongue; Salami; Bologna; Chicken skin; Chorizo; Frankfurters; Lamb tongue; Luncheon meats; Pepperoni; Pork breakfast strips; Pork ribs; Pork skins; Pork spare ribs; Sausages; Turkey skins; Pork headcheese; Pork liver cheese; Pastrami; Lamb ribs; Pork shoulder; Organ Meats; Beef chuck/brisket; Beef (ground); Corned beef; Beef ribs; Pork back ribs; Lamb; Goose; Cured Meats; Pork; Beef shank; Chicken wings; Game Meat; Bison/buffalo meat; Chicken dark meat; Squab (pigeon); Beef; Quail; Frog legs; Boar meat; Rabbit meat; Abalone; Goat meat; Croaker; Veal; Venison; Caribou meat; Duck (no skin); Eel; Whelk;

Instead Choose: Crayfish; Cuttlefish; Shrimp; Pheasant; Turkey dark meat; Guinea hen; Squid (Calamari); Beef filet mignon;

Eggs, Beans, Nuts and Seeds

Egg yolk; Pili nuts; Brazil nuts; Butternuts; Pine nuts; Hickory nuts; Seeds: watermelon, pumpkin/squash, cottonseed, safflower, sesame; Cashew nuts; Beechnuts; Pecans; Walnuts (black); Peanuts; Almonds; Coconut meat (dried); Pistachio nuts; Walnuts; Seeds (sunflower); Coconut meat (raw); Hazelnuts or Filberts; Acorns; Egg (hard-boiled); Egg (raw); Egg (duck); Soy milk; Coconut milk; Cornnuts; Macadamia nuts; Chestnuts; Soybeans (green); Ginkgo nuts; Breadfruit seeds;

Instead Choose: Chickpeas; Beans (baked); Seeds (breadnut tree); Egg white;

Fruits & Juices

Tamarind; Prune juice; Avocado; Limit consumption of fruit juices;

Instead Choose: Apples (dried); Cherries; Figs (dried); Raisins; Orange juice; Figs; Quince; Longans (dried); Grapes; Litchi; Litchi (dried); Grapefruit juice; Cranberry juice; Currants (dried); Dates; Pears (dried); Apple juice; Pineapple juice; Plantains; Longans; Grape juice; Pomegranate juice;

Breads, Grains, Cereals, Pasta

Cereal (wheat germ); Biscuits; Bread (banana); Bread (cornbread); Cereal (granola); Croissant; Donuts; Granola bars; Various Muffins; Sweet rolls; Waffles; Crackers (wheat); Bread sticks; Noodles (Chinese chow Mein); Rolls (whole-wheat dinner); Danish pastry; Cereals; Rolls (Kaiser); Crackers (milk); Melba toast; Crackers (whole-wheat); Wheat germ; Rolls (hamburger/hot dog); Bread (Italian); Crackers (saltines); Toasted bread; Bagels; Bread (white); Bread (oat bran); Cereal (whole-wheat); English muffins; Rolls (French); Bread (wheat germ); Wheat; Bread (French/Sourdough); Whole-wheat; English muffins (whole-wheat); Cereal (shredded wheat); Rice (white); Cereal (cream of wheat); Bulgur; Bread (pumpernickel); Bread (whole-wheat); Spaghetti; Couscous; Noodles (egg); Spaghetti (whole-wheat); Crackers (matzo); Spelt; Rice cakes (Brown rice); Durum wheat; Semolina; Tortillas (corn); Corn; Amaranth; Millet; Wheat bran; Noodles (rice); Rice (wild);

Instead *Choose*: ***Rice bran; Rye grain; Quinoa; Oat bran; Oats; Sorghum grain; Barley; Spaghetti (spinach); Noodles (Japanese); Oatmeal (cereal); Pasta;***

Dairy Products, Fats & Oils

Butter; Various Cheese; Cheese spread; Cream (whipped); Hydrogenated vegetable oil; Margarine; Margarine-like spreads; Non-dairy creamers; Oils: cottonseed, wheat germ; Vegetable shortening; Fat (chicken, duck, turkey); Lard; Oils: (palm, tea seed, corn, poppy seed, sesame, tomato seeds; Other Oils; Milk (chocolate); Milk (whole); Fat (beef/lamb/pork); Sour cream; Milk (skim); Milk (1% fat); Milk (2% fat); Oil (canola); Buttermilk; Whey (sweet); Cream; Cheese (Cottage);

Instead *Choose*: ***Oil (olive);***

Desserts, Snacks, Beverages

Sherbet; After-dinner mints; Brownies; Cakes; Candies; Cheesecake; Chewing gum; Chocolate mousse; Coffee liqueur; Coffeecake; Cookies; Cream puffs/Éclair; Crème de menthe; Dessert toppings; Frostings; Fruit leather/rolls; Halvah (candy); Honey; Ice creams; Ice cream cones; Jams & Preserves; Jellies; Marshmallows; Peanut butter; Pies; Pie crust; Popcorn (oil popped); Potato sticks; Puff pastry; Taro chips; Tortilla chips; Frozen yogurt; Molasses; Chocolate (sweet); Milk shakes; Chocolate (dark); Pancakes; Potato chips; Eggnog; Pudding; Applesauce; Piña colada; Ginger ale; Hot chocolate; Tonic water; Pretzels; Fruit punch; Lemonade; Soft (carbonated) drinks; Popcorn (air popped); Red Bull (drink); Sports drinks; 80+ proof distilled alc. bev.; Whiskey; Malted drinks (nonalcoholic); Coffee; Tea (plain); Wine (red); Wine (white); Beer;

Instead *Choose*: ***Coffee (decaf); Tea (herbal); Beer;***

Herbs & Spices, Fast Foods, Prepared Foods

Breaded shrimp; Cheeseburger; Foie gras or liver pate; French toast; Hash brown potatoes; Hush puppies; Nachos; Onion rings; Pizza; Potato pancakes; Salad dressings; Syrup (chocolate); Taco shells; Tahini; Syrup (maple); Hot dog; Syrup (sorghum); Hamburger; Syrup (table blends); Potato salad; Sausage (meatless); Teriyaki sauce; French fries; Sugar (brown); Sugar (table, powder); Chicken Nuggets; Soy sauce; Tofu (fried); Syrup (malt); Hummus; Corn cakes; Barbecue sauce; Egg rolls (veg); Natto; Mayonnaise; Sauce (Hoisin); Cottonseed meal; Pickle (sweet); Ketchup; Sauce (fish); Falafel; Sauce (oyster); Tofu; Beef broth & stock; Sauces; Sugar (maple); Macaroni; Chicken broth; Tabasco sauce; Cornmeal (whole-grain); Tempeh; Cole slaw; Chicken stock; Croutons; Poppy seed; Salt (table); Cocoa;

Instead Choose: *Rosemary (fresh); Corn salad; Parsley; Succotash; Dill weed; Miso; Herbs & Spices; Tomato paste; Balsamic vinegar; Gravies; Horseradish; Pickle; Vinegar; Sauerkraut; Mustard; Soups: veg/beef, chicken noodle, beef barley; Kimchi; Capers;*

Alternative Therapies & Miscellaneous

Corn syrup; Deep-fried foods; 2+ alcoholic drinks/day; Artificial sweeteners; Tapioca pearls; Saccharine (NutraSweet); Aspartame (Equal); Cheese made w/whole milk; Baking using butter; Excessive TV viewing (avoid eating while watching); Food additives/preservatives (choose fresh food, limit packaged food); Smoked fish/food; Processed or Refined foods; Skipping meals; Stress; Artificial colors; BHA (butylated hydroxyanisole); BHT (butylated hydroxytoluene); FD&C yellow dye #5. Tartrazine; Food additives Nitrates/Nitrites; Monosodium Glutamate; Pesticide-loaded crops; Sulfite (preservative); Waxes (preservative for fruits and vegs); Smoking/Tobacco; Canned foods; Toasted bread/foods; Salted foods, nuts, etc.;

Key Nutrients & Herbal Meds

Trans fatty acids; Omega-6 fatty acid (LA); Fat (saturated); Sugar (refined); Carbohydrates; Cholesterol; Sugar (total); Limit calorie consumption per day to 10 per pound of desired weight;

Depression (& HT)

Depression is a serious chronic illness. It is not just a temporary feeling of being down. It is a disorder of the brain. It can interfere with your normal life and lead to various physical and emotional problems. It affects men, women and elderly in different ways.

The exact cause of depression is unknown. But several factors can lead to depression: loss of a loved one, stressful situations such as a difficult relationship or financial problems, family history of depression (genetic factors), differences in brain chemistry, changes in body hormones, and traumatic events during one's childhood.

You are more likely to get depression if you are between 15 and 30 years old, you are a woman, it is winter time, or it is just after you gave birth to a baby.

Choose these for Depression & HT

Top 5 items to consume:

Fish; Shellfish; Soybeans; Garlic; Fish Oil; & Exercise

Food items and actions that could improve your health (within a food group, most helpful items are listed first):

Meat, Fish & Poultry

Anchovy; **Bluefish**; **Cisco (smoked)**; **Mackerel**; **Mackerel (king)**; **Marlin**; **Salmon (pink)**; **Spot**; **Sturgeon**; **Swordfish**; **Trout**; **Tuna (blue fin)**; **White fish**; **Herring**; **Sablefish**; **Tilefish**; **Salmon (smoked, Lox)**; **Mussels**; **Caviar**; **Bass (striped)**; **Smelt**; **Tuna (yellowfin)**; **Halibut**; **Bass (seabass)**; **Wolffish**; **Pollock**; **Sucker**; **Mullet**; **Bass (freshwater)**; **Drum**; **Whiting**; **Shad**; **Lobster (spiny)**; **Crab (Dungeness)**; **Milkfish**; **Yellowtail**; **Cisco**; **Surimi**; **Oysters**; **Pompano fish**; **Crab (snow)**; **Tilapia**; **Clams**; **Dolphinfish (Mahi-Mahi)**; **Seatrout**; **Walleye**; **Crab (Alaskan King)**; **Octopus**; **White fish (smoked)**; **Grouper**; **Snapper**; **Flatfish (flounder & sole)**; **Butterfish**; **Scup**; **Catfish**; **Lingcod**; **Burbot**; **Rockfish**; **Cusk**; **Chicken breast (no skin)**; **Carp**; **Perch**; **Haddock**; **Northern pike**; **Cod**; **Ling**; **Sheepshead**; **Monkfish**; **Pumpkinseed sunfish**; **Turbot**; **Conch**; **Pout**; **Cuttlefish**; **Orange roughy**; **Turkey breast**; **Sardines**; Lobster; Turkey dark meat; Whelk; Caribou meat; Fish roe; Shark; Crab (Blue); Tuna (canned); Shrimp; Veal; Snail; Scallops; Squid (Calamari); Pheasant breast; Beef filet mignon; Crayfish; Quail breast; Venison; Lamb leg; Liver; Eel; Rabbit meat; Goat meat; Beef rib eye; Pheasant; Beef round steak; Beef top sirloin; Lamb & Pork kidneys; Beef tenderloin/T-bone/porterhouse; Croaker; Boar meat; Guinea hen;

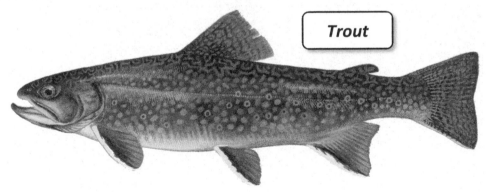

Trout

Eggs, Beans, Nuts and Seeds

Soybeans (dried); **Seeds (flaxseed)**; **Peas (sugar/snap)**; **Peas (green)**; **Seeds (chia)**; Lentils; Beans: black, moth beans, navy, pinto; Black-eyed peas; Other Beans; Egg white; Peas (split); Pigeon peas; Alfalfa sprouts; Seeds (breadnut tree); Ginkgo nuts; Breadfruit seeds; Soybeans (green); Lupin; Chickpeas; Egg substitute; Macadamia nuts; Egg (duck); Chestnuts; Cornnuts;

Fruits & Juices

Guava; Acerola; Lemon; Orange juice; Pumelo (Shaddock); Strawberries; Currants (raw); Jujube (fruit); Kiwi fruit; Oranges; Papaya; Durian; Natal Plum (Carissa); Elderberries; Pineapple; Mango; Persimmons; Abiyuch; Boysenberries; Lime; Starfruit; Cantaloupe; Grapefruit juice; Berries; Olives; Rhubarb; Kumquats; Pitanga; Passion fruit; Grapefruit; Banana; Litchi; Apple juice; Apricots; Nectarine; Peaches; Plum; Watermelon; Litchi (dried); Longans; Apples; Cranberry juice; Grape juice; Pomegranate juice; Pears; Prunes (dried); Honeydew melon; Pineapple juice; Tangerines; Breadfruit; Dried Fruits; Cherries; Pomegranate; Raisins; Prune juice; Rowal; Plantains; Dates; Figs; Grapes; Tamarind; Quince; **Avoid sugared and made from concentrate juices;**

Vegetables

Garlic; **Winged beans leaves**; **Peppers (jalapeno)**; **Peppers (pimento)**; **Arrowroot**; **Taro leaves**; **Artichoke**; **Peppers (hot chili)**; **Kelp**; **Broccoli**; **Mushrooms (shitake)**; Amaranth leaves; Balsam pear leafy tips; Collards; Cowpeas leafy tips; Epazote; Garden cress; Kale; Lambsquarters; Mustard spinach; Peppers (pasilla); Sesbania Flower; Spinach; Turnip greens; Vine spinach (Basella); Brussels sprouts; Chrysanthemum (Garland); Chrysanthemum Leaves; Bell peppers (red); Taro (Tahitian); Cauliflower; Grape leaves; Mustard greens; Dandelion Greens; Mushrooms; Chicory greens; Balsam pear; Bok choy; Cabbage (savoy); Peppers; Pokeberry shoots; Endive; Bell peppers (green); Broccoli (Chinese); Cabbage (red); Kohlrabi; Asparagus; Okra; Squash (Acorn); Arugula; Cabbage (green); Lettuce (Romaine); Onions; Beet greens; Borage; Pumpkin flowers; Swiss chard; Watercress; Potato; Sweet potatoes leaves; Tomatoes (sun-dried); Potatoes w/skin; Yam; Parsnips; Celtuce; Green onions (scallions); Leeks; Purslane; Beets; Other Vegetables;

Breads, Grains, Cereals, Pasta

Bread (French/Sourdough); English muffins (whole-wheat); Cereal (corn flakes); Bread (wheat germ); Bread (whole-wheat); Oats; Buckwheat; Triticale; Toasted bread; Rice bran; Durum wheat; Whole-wheat; Rice (brown); Cereal (rice crisps); Spelt; Rye grain; Cereal (whole-wheat); Bread (Italian); Spaghetti (whole-wheat); Quinoa; Sorghum grain; Cereal (raisin bran); Barley; Wheat bran; Oatmeal (cereal); Rice (wild); Bread (oat bran); Rice cakes (Brown rice); Cereal (bran flakes); Millet; Amaranth; Bulgur; Corn; Bread (pumpernickel); Pasta; Spaghetti; Cereal (shredded wheat);

Dairy Products, Fats & Oils

Fish oil (salmon); **Fish oil (cod liver)**; **Other Fish oil**; Oil (flaxseed); Cheese (Cottage);

Desserts, Snacks, Beverages

Water (eight cups of fluid daily); Tea (green);

Herbs & Spices, Fast Foods, Prepared Foods

Ginger; Soup (clam chowder); Miso; Cornmeal (whole-grain); Fish stock; Tofu; Tempeh; Cottonseed meal; Cayenne (red) pepper; Cinnamon; Corn salad; Kimchi; Thyme (fresh);

Alternative Therapies & Miscellaneous

Exercise (including cardiovascular, weight training, walking, biking or jogging); Wild fish and free range animals; Fresh (uncooked) fruits/veg's; Socialize, join a club; Organic cold-pressed oils;

Key Nutrients & Herbal Meds

Omega-3 fatty acids; Vitamin B-3 (Niacin; in nicotinic acid form, not recommended as supplement or drug); DHEA (dehydroepiandosterone); Folic Acid (deficiency could be the cause for depression); Ginkgo Biloba; SAMe (works best with vitamin B12 and folic acid); St. John's wort (dose of 2-4 grams of the herb for a mild antidepressant action or nervous disturbances); Valerian (don't combine with alcohol);

Do not choose these for Depression & HT

Top 5 items to avoid:

> Sweets; Luncheon Meats; Fast Foods; Salad Dressings; Vegetable Shortening;

Avoid or consume much less of the following (within a food group, most harmful items are listed first):

Meat, Fish & Poultry

Bologna; **Frankfurters**; **Pepperoni**; **Sausages**; **Salami**; **Bacon**; **Luncheon meats**; **Chorizo**; **Pork breakfast strips**; **Pastrami**; **Chicken skin**; **Beef (cured brkfst strips)**; **Turkey skins**; **Pork skins**; **Beef tongue**; **Pork spare ribs**; **Beef jerky sticks**; **Pork liver cheese**; **Goose**; **Pork ribs**; **Corned beef**; Pork headcheese; Pork shoulder; Cured Meats; Beef (ground); Chicken wings; Organ meats; Beef chuck/brisket; Lamb ribs; Beef ribs; Pork back ribs; Chicken dark meat; Beef shank; Squab (pigeon); Quail; Lamb (ground);

Instead **Choose**: Abalone; Pork loin/sirloin; Bison/buffalo meat; Duck (no skin); Veal kidneys; Lamb loin & shoulder;

Eggs, Beans, Nuts and Seeds

Pine nuts; **Coconut meat (dried)**; **Butternuts**; Hickory nuts; Pili nuts; Brazil nuts; Seeds (watermelon); Beechnuts; Pecans; Seeds: sesame, pumpkin/squash; Cashew nuts; Pistachio nuts; Walnuts (black); Seeds: safflower, cottonseed; Almonds; Walnuts; Peanuts; Hazelnuts or Filberts; Soy milk; Coconut milk; Coconut meat (raw); Acorns; Seeds (sunflower);

Instead **Choose**: Egg (hard-boiled); Egg (raw); Egg yolk;

Breads, Grains, Cereals, Pasta

Danish pastry; **Donuts**; **Muffins (blueberry)**; **Sweet rolls**; **Granola bars**; **Cereal (granola)**; **Crackers (wheat)**; **Muffins: wheat bran, oat bran**; **Crackers (milk)**; **Croissant**; **Bread (cornbread)**; **Bread (banana)**; **Waffles**; **Biscuits**; Muffins (corn); Crackers (whole-wheat); Rolls (whole-wheat dinner); Crackers (saltines); Noodles (Chinese chow Mein); Rolls (Kaiser); Noodles (egg); Cereal (cream of wheat); Bread sticks; Melba toast; Crackers (matzo); Cereal (wheat germ); Wheat germ; Rolls (hamburger/hot dog); Tortillas (corn); Bread (white);

Instead **Choose**: Spaghetti (spinach); Semolina; Oat bran; Rolls (French); Bagels; Wheat; Couscous; English muffins; Noodles (Japanese); Rice (white); Noodles (rice);

Dairy Products, Fats & Oils

Margarine-like spreads; Non-dairy creamers; Vegetable shortening; Oils: cottonseed, corn, poppy seed, sesame, tomato seeds, grape seeds, walnut; Milk (chocolate); Fat (chicken, turkey); Other Oils; Butter; Fat (duck); Lard; Cheese (American); Hydrogenated vegetable oil; Margarine; Cheese (Cream); Cream (whipped); Milk (whole); Fat (beef/lamb/pork); Cheese (Cheddar); Cheese spread; Cheese (Pimento); Cheese (Colby); Other Cheese; Milk (skim); Buttermilk; Sour cream; Milk (1% fat); Milk; Milk (2% fat); Whey (sweet); Cream; Yogurt;

Instead Choose: Oil (olive);

Desserts, Snacks, Beverages

Brownies; Cakes; Candies; Chocolate mousse; Coffee liqueur; Coffeecake; Cookies; Cream puffs/Éclair; Crème de menthe; Dessert toppings; Frostings; Ice cream (chocolate); Pies; Puff pastry; Taro chips; Cheesecake; After-dinner mints; Fruit leather/rolls; Carob (candy); Chewing gum; Pudding; Ice cream (vanilla); Frozen yogurt; Chocolate (sweet); Potato sticks; Halvah (candy); Sherbet; Jams & Preserves; Jellies; Marshmallows; Honey; Peanut butter; Tortilla chips; Piña colada; Potato chips; Soft (carbonated) drinks; Hot chocolate; Pie crust; Milk shakes; Eggnog; Chocolate; Applesauce; Molasses; 80+ proof distilled alc. bev.; Fruit punch; Lemonade; Whiskey; Pancakes; Ginger ale; Tonic water; Popcorn (oil popped); Ice cream cones; Sports drinks; Wine (red); Wine (white); Coffee; Tea (plain); Beer; Chocolate (dark); Popcorn (air popped); Malted drinks (nonalcoholic);

Instead Choose: Pretzels; Coffee (decaf); Tea (herbal); Red Bull (drink);

Herbs & Spices, Fast Foods, Prepared Foods

Nachos; Onion rings; Salad dressings; Syrup (chocolate); Pizza; Hush puppies; Breaded shrimp; Sugar (table, powder); Syrup (table blends); Hot dog; Potato salad; Teriyaki sauce; Hash brown potatoes; Syrup (maple); Sugar (brown); Syrup (sorghum); Barbecue sauce; Mayonnaise; Sausage (meatless); Taco shells; French toast; Chicken Nuggets; Natto; Hummus; French fries; Tahini; Sauce (Hoisin); Cheeseburger; Foie gras or liver pate; Potato pancakes; Egg rolls (veg); Ketchup; Soy sauce; Pickle (sweet); Hamburger; Syrup (malt); Sauces; Tofu (fried); Poppy seed; Macaroni; Sugar (maple); Cocoa; Chicken broth; Soup (chicken noodle); Chicken stock;

Instead Choose: Succotash; Croutons; Mints; Parsley; Falafel; Dill weed; Sauerkraut; Balsamic vinegar; Herbs & Spices; Capers; Gravies; Horseradish; Mustard; Pickle; Salt (table); Tomato paste; Vinegar; Soups: veg/beef, beef barley; Cole slaw;

Alternative Therapies & Miscellaneous

Corn syrup; Deep-fried foods; 2+ alcoholic drinks/day; Smoking/Tobacco; Artificial sweeteners (e.g., sorbitol, mannitol, xylitol, maltitol and isomaltose); Cheese made w/whole milk; Excess body weight; Aspartame (Equal); Saccharine (NutraSweet); Processed or Refined foods; Birth control pills; Prescription drugs; 1-2 alcoholic drinks/day; Baking using butter; Stress;

Key Nutrients & Herbal Meds

Trans fatty acids; Omega-6 fatty acid (LA); Alcohol; Sugar (refined); Fat (saturated); Marijuana;

Alzheimer's Disease (& HT)

Dementia is a brain disorder that refers to our loss of ability to think, remember, reason and perform daily activities. Among people older than 60, Alzheimer's Disease (AD) is the most common cause of dementia.

AD causes the gradual decline and loss of brain cells and the ability for cells (neuron) to communicate with each other. Thus a person affected with AD, has fewer brain cells and fewer connections among the brain's remaining cells. This results in a steady decline in our memory (as In remembering people's names, or doing daily tasks), and cognitive functions such as reasoning.

A combination of factors is believed to cause AD. Among these risk factors are: age (starting at the age of 60 and increasing over time), immediate family history of AD, sex (women are more likely than men to develop AD), and the same risk factors associated with heart disease (i.e., high blood pressure, high cholesterol, diabetes, lack of exercise and smoking). Higher levels of on-going intellectual and social activities have been found to reduce the risk of developing AD.

There is neither a proven approach to prevent nor to cure this disease. But there has been a 2015 study conducted by the scientists at the Rush University, whereby a combination of the Mediterranean diet and DASH (Dietary Approaches to Stop Hypertension) diet, known as the MIND diet, has shown that this diet can lower the risk of AD significantly. There has also been some evidence that reducing risk of high blood pressure, high cholesterol, obesity and diabetes can reduce the risk of developing AD. Therefore, proper nutrition, exercise and staying mentally and socially active can all play an important role.

Choose these for Alzheimer's Disease & HT

Top 5 items to consume:

**Fish; Fish Oil; Garlic & Artichoke; Shellfish;
Green Tea; & Exercise;**

Food items and actions that could improve your health (within a food group, most helpful items are listed first):

Meat, Fish & Poultry

Anchovy; **Bluefish**; **Cisco (smoked)**; **Mackerel**; **Marlin**; **Salmon (pink)**; **Spot**; **Sturgeon**; **Swordfish**; **Trout**; **Tuna (blue fin)**; **White fish**; **Herring**; **Sablefish**; **Tilefish**; **Mackerel (king)**; **Bass (striped)**; **Smelt**; **Halibut**; **Bass (seabass)**; **Wolffish**; **Pollock**; **Sucker**; **Bass (freshwater)**; **Drum**; **Whiting**; **Tuna (yellowfin)**; **Caviar**; **Mullet**; **Pompano fish**; **Shad**; **Salmon (smoked, Lox)**; **Cisco**; **Surimi**; **Walleye**; **Seatrout**; **Snapper**; **Mussels**; **Catfish**; **Milkfish**; **White fish (smoked)**; **Carp**; **Tilapia**; **Yellowtail**; **Rockfish**; **Oysters**; **Grouper**; **Perch**; **Flatfish (flounder & sole)**; **Dolphinfish (Mahi-Mahi)**; **Burbot**; **Lingcod**; **Lobster (spiny)**; **Scup**; **Butterfish**; **Cusk**; **Crab (Dungeness)**; **Northern pike**; **Chicken breast (no skin)**; Ling; Cod; Sheepshead; Haddock; Pumpkinseed sunfish; Monkfish; Orange roughy; Pout; Crab (snow); Fish roe; Sardines; Pheasant breast; Turbot; Conch; Crab (Alaskan King); Octopus; Shark; Quail breast; Snail; Eel; Turkey dark meat; Turkey breast; Clams; Lobster; Pheasant; Tuna (canned); Guinea hen; Cuttlefish; Squid (Calamari); Crab (Blue); Crayfish; Whelk; Scallops; Shrimp; Duck (no skin);

Eggs, Beans, Nuts and Seeds

Soybeans (dried); Peas (sugar/snap); Macadamia nuts; Peas (green); Ginkgo nuts; Breadfruit seeds; Lentils; Beans (yardlong); Alfalfa sprouts; Beans/Legumes (1+ servings every other day for AD); Beans: hyacinth, moth beans, mung; Peas (split); Seeds: flaxseed, chia; Other Beans; Pigeon peas; Chestnuts; Black-eyed peas; Nuts (5+ servings/week for AD); Cornnuts; Lupin; Egg white;

Fruits & Juices

Blueberries; Elderberries; Mulberries; Cranberries; Various Berries (2+ servings/week for AD); Cranberry juice; Pomegranate; Acerola; Lemon; Orange juice; Pumelo (Shaddock); Currants (raw); Guava; Jujube (fruit); Kiwi fruit; Oranges; Papaya; Grapes; Natal Plum (Carissa); Pineapple; Persimmons; Abiyuch; Lime; Starfruit; Cantaloupe; Grapefruit juice; **Avoid sugared or made from concentrate juices;**

Vegetables (green leafy vegetables or a salad, and one other vegetable everyday)

Garlic; **Artichoke**; **Winged beans leaves**; **Peppers (jalapeno)**; **Peppers (pimento)**; **Chicory greens**; **Taro leaves**; **Fiddlehead ferns**; **Mushrooms (Chanterelle)**; **Peppers (hot chili)**; **Broccoli**; **Peppers (hot chili, red)**; Amaranth leaves; Arugula; Balsam pear leafy tips; Beet greens; Bell peppers (green); Broccoli (Chinese); Brussels sprouts; Cabbage (green); Collards; Dandelion Greens; Epazote; Garden cress; Kale; Lambsquarters; Various Lettuce; Mustard greens; Mustard spinach; Okra; Peppers; Spinach; Sweet potatoes leaves; Swiss chard; Turnip greens; Vine spinach (Basella); Watercress; Green onions (scallions); Zucchini; Mushrooms (shitake); Taro (Tahitian); Grape leaves; Chrysanthemum Leaves; Cauliflower; Asparagus; Bell peppers (red); Celery; Green beans; Mushrooms (portabella); Cabbage (red); Kohlrabi; Onions; Balsam pear; Pokeberry shoots; Sesbania Flower; Cowpeas leafy tips; Bok choy; Mushrooms (Morel); Borage; Squash (Acorn); Cabbage (savoy); Other Vegetables;

Breads, Grains, Cereals, Pasta

Oats; Triticale; Buckwheat; Durum wheat; Sorghum grain; Whole-wheat; Rye grain; Whole Grains (3+ servings/day); Rice (brown); Millet; Spelt; Barley; Corn; Cereal (whole-wheat); Oatmeal (cereal); Wheat bran; Spaghetti (whole-wheat); English muffins (whole-wheat); Bulgur; Rice (wild); Amaranth; Quinoa; Rice bran;

Dairy Products, Fats & Oils

Fish oil (cod liver); **Fish oil (salmon)**; **Other Fish oils**; **Oil (olive, use as your primary oil at home)**; Oil (flaxseed);

Desserts, Snacks, Beverages

Tea (green); Red Bull (drink); Wine (one glass of wine/day for AD); Coffee; Tea (plain);

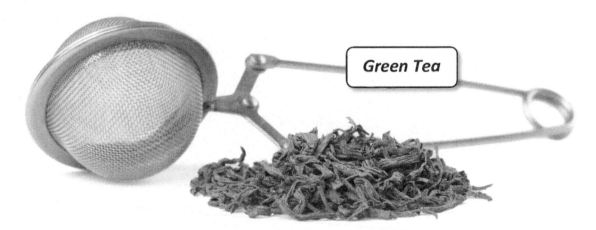

Green Tea

Herbs & Spices, Fast Foods, Prepared Foods

Cinnamon; Ginger; Parsley; Thyme (fresh); Cocoa; Turmeric; Fish stock; Basil (fresh); Coriander/Cilantro; Mints; Peppermint; Rosemary (fresh); Spearmint (fresh); Cayenne (red) pepper; Soup (clam chowder); Corn salad;

Alternative Therapies & Miscellaneous

Exercise (i.e., Cardiovascular, Weight Training, walking, jogging, or cycling); Wild fish and free range animals; Challenge your mind (puzzles, games, books); Mediterranean diet; Exposure to sun; Green plants and vegetables;

Key Nutrients & Herbal Meds

Omega-3 fatty acids; Chlorophyll; Vitamin B-3 (Niacin, in nicotinic acid form, not recommended as supplement or drug);

Do not choose these for Alzheimer's Disease & HT

Top 5 items to avoid:

Luncheon/Processed Meats; Cheese; Hydrogenated Vegetable Oil; Fast Foods; Sweets;

Avoid or consume much less of the following (within a food group, most harmful items are listed first):

Meat, Fish & Poultry

Bacon; Beef (cured brkfst strips); Salami; Bologna; Chorizo; Frankfurters; Pepperoni; Pork breakfast strips; Pork skins; Sausages; Luncheon meats; Pork liver cheese; Pastrami; Pork spare ribs; Beef jerky sticks; Pork headcheese; Pork ribs; Beef tongue; Lamb ribs; Veal heart; Pork shoulder; Organ meats; Corned beef; Beef chuck/brisket; Beef (cured dried); Beef (ground); Cured Meats; Turkey & Chicken skins; Pork; Lamb; Beef ribs; Beaver meat; Beef shank; Bear meat; Bison/buffalo meat; Frog legs; Beef; Boar meat; Chicken wings; Goat meat; Goose; Rabbit meat; Venison; Veal shoulder; Chicken dark meat; Caribou meat; Beef filet mignon; Veal shank; Abalone; Veal loin; Squab (pigeon);

Instead Choose: Croaker; Quail;

Eggs, Beans, Nuts and Seeds

Seeds: safflower, cottonseed, watermelon, sesame, pumpkin/squash; Coconut meat (dried); Egg yolk; Seeds (sunflower); Egg (hard-boiled); Soy milk; Egg (raw); Butternuts; Pili nuts; Coconut milk; Beechnuts; Brazil nuts; Hickory nuts; Pine nuts; Pistachio nuts; Egg (duck); Cashew nuts; Peanuts; Coconut meat (raw); Walnuts (black); Pecans; Almonds; Acorns;

Instead Choose: Egg substitute; Seeds (breadnut tree); Hazelnuts or Filberts; Beans (baked); Beans (winged); Soybeans (green); Walnuts; Chickpeas;

Fruits & Juices

Avocado; Tamarind; Longans (dried); Plantains; Quince; **Avoid sugared or made from concentrate juices;**

Instead Choose: Olives; Rhubarb; Kumquats; Pitanga; Grapefruit; Mango; Peaches; Passion fruit; Litchi; Apple juice; Apricots; Nectarine; Plum; Watermelon; Grape juice; Durian; Apples; Longans; Pears; Pomegranate juice; Honeydew melon; Pineapple juice; Banana; Tangerines; Raisins; Breadfruit; Cherries; Dried fruits; Rowal; Dates; Prune juice; Figs;

Breads, Grains, Cereals, Pasta

Donuts; **Muffins (blueberry)**; **Danish pastry**; **Sweet rolls**; **Biscuits**; **Bread (cornbread)**; **Muffins (oat bran)**; **Croissant**; **Waffles**; **Muffins (wheat bran)**; **Granola bars**; **Bread sticks**; **Bread (banana)**; **Crackers (wheat)**; **Muffins (corn)**; **Noodles (Chinese chow Mein)**; **Cereal (granola)**; **Rolls (Kaiser)**; **Crackers (milk)**; **Rolls (whole-wheat dinner)**; Cereal (wheat germ); Melba toast; Crackers (whole-wheat); Rolls (hamburger/hot dog); Crackers (saltines); Bread (white); Bread (Italian); Bread (pumpernickel); Rolls (French); Cereal (bran flakes); Tortillas (corn); Wheat germ; English muffins; Bagels; Cereal (raisin bran); Toasted bread; Bread (oat bran); Cereal (shredded wheat); Noodles (egg); Cereal (cream of wheat); Bread (French/Sourdough); Cereal (rice crisps); Bread (wheat germ); Cereal (corn flakes); Crackers (matzo); Pasta;

Instead <u>*Choose*</u>*: Bread (whole-wheat); Rice cakes (Brown rice); Spaghetti (spinach); Oat bran; Cornmeal (whole-grain); Croutons; Semolina; Noodles (Japanese); Couscous; Noodles (rice); Wheat; Rice (white); Spaghetti;*

Dairy Products, Fats & Oils

Various Cheese (limit to less than one serving per week); **Cheese spread**; **Hydrogenated vegetable oil**; **Vegetable shortening**; **Butter (less than 1 TBS of butter or margarine/day)**; **Margarine-like spreads**; **Non-dairy creamers**; **Margarine (less than 1 TBS of butter or margarine/day)**; **Oils: cottonseed, Ucuhuba Butter, sesame, tomato seeds**; **Fat (chicken, turkey, duck)**; **Other Oils**; **Lard**; **Cream (whipped)**; **Milk (whole)**; **Cheese (Cottage)**; Fat (beef/lamb/pork); Sour cream; Milk (chocolate); Milk (skim); Oil (canola); Milk (1% fat); Milk (2% fat); Buttermilk; Oil (coconut); Whey (sweet); Cream; Yogurt;

Desserts, Snacks, Beverages

Dessert toppings; **Cakes**; **Candies**; **Pies**; **Pie crust**; **Puff pastry**; **Cookies**; **Brownies**; **Cheesecake**; **Frostings**; **Coffeecake**; **Ice cream cones**; **After-dinner mints**; **Cream puffs/Éclair**; **Halvah (candy)**; **Ice cream (vanilla)**; **Chocolate mousse**; **Sherbet**; **Chewing gum**; **Jams & Preserves**; **Jellies**; **Candies (hard)**; **Marshmallows**; **Frozen yogurt**; **Taro chips**; **Ice cream (chocolate)**; **Pancakes**; **Potato sticks**; **Tortilla chips**; **Pudding**; **Potato chips**; **Fruit leather/rolls**; **Chocolate (sweet)**; **Pretzels**; **Peanut butter**; **Popcorn (oil popped)**; Crème de menthe; Honey; Milk shakes; Coffee liqueur; Piña colada; Eggnog; Popcorn (air popped); Molasses; Applesauce; Soft (carbonated) drinks; Ginger ale; Tonic water; 80+ proof distilled alc. bev.; Fruit punch; Lemonade; Whiskey; Sports drinks; Malted drinks (nonalcoholic); Hot chocolate; Chocolate (dark);

Instead <u>*Choose*</u>*: Coffee (decaf); Tea (herbal); Water; Beer;*

Herbs & Spices, Fast Foods, Prepared Foods

Breaded shrimp; Cheeseburger; Hush puppies; Nachos; Onion rings; Pizza; Hot dog; French fries; Hamburger; Salad dressings; Teriyaki sauce; Fast foods (limit to less than one serving per week); Potato salad; Taco shells; Hash brown potatoes; French toast; Sausage (meatless); Soy sauce; Potato pancakes; Egg rolls (veg); Foie gras or liver pate; Hummus; Mayonnaise; Chicken Nuggets; Natto; Tahini; Syrup (chocolate); Syrup (maple); Tofu (fried); Syrup (table blends); Beef broth & stock; Soups: veg/beef, beef barley; Sugar (table, powder); Syrup (sorghum); Sugar (brown); Cottonseed meal; Barbecue sauce; Tempeh; Corn cakes; Tofu; Chicken broth; Soup (chicken noodle); Sauces; Poppy seed; Salt (table); Chicken stock; Syrup (malt); Sugar (maple); Ketchup; Pickle (sweet); Macaroni; Miso; Sauerkraut;

Instead <u>Choose</u>*: Dill weed; Succotash; Cornmeal (whole-grain); Balsamic vinegar; Herbs & Spices; Gravies; Horseradish; Pickle; Tomato paste; Vinegar; Cole slaw; Kimchi; Falafel; Mustard; Soups: minestrone, tomato, vegetable; Sauces: cheese, hot, tomato; Capers*

Alternative Therapies & Miscellaneous

Deep-fried foods (limit to less than one serving/week for AD); Smoking/Tobacco; Cheese made w/whole milk; Excess body weight; Stress; Corn syrup; 2+ alcoholic drinks/day; Canned foods; Artificial sweeteners; Baking using butter;

Key Nutrients & Herbal Meds

Omega-6 fatty acid (LA); Trans fatty acids; Fat (saturated);

Cancer Risk (& HT)

Cells are the building block of every organ in our body. Cells reproduce or die at varying rates depending on the organ and our age. Sometimes we have abnormal cells that reproduce or divide at a faster rate than we need. This phenomenon results in a collection of unwanted cells called a tumor. If the cells in the tumor have the ability to infiltrate other tissues and organs in our body then this tumor is considered malignant, otherwise it is considered benign. Cancer is the condition that corresponds to the malignant tumors. Cancer refers to as many as 200 different diseases but they all have the out of control cell reproduction in common.

Cancers are named after the organ where a tumor first appears. Some cancers do not form a tumor such as cancer of blood. In medical jargon, if cancer affects soft tissues and organs such as breast or lung, they are categorized as Carcinomas. If cancer affects hard tissues such as bone or muscle, they are called Sarcomas. If cancer affects our lymphatic system (i.e., part of body's circulatory system which transports things such as plasma, fats, white cells from one place to another throughout our body), it is called Lymphoma. And finally if cancer affects tissues such as blood or bone marrow, it is known as Leukemia.

There has been significant progress in cancer research and treatment of cancer over the recent decades. We understand that gene mutations are the cause of cancer development. We also know of most of the causes for gene mutations that cause cancer, i.e., the carcinogens. In short, the research has led to identification of various risk factors that increase the possibility of developing cancer. The most common of which are: family history of cancer; age (growing older); exposure to Ultraviolet (UV) radiation (from sun, tanning booths, sunlamps); certain infections; hormones (e.g., estrogen); exposure to certain chemicals (e.g., radon gas, asbestos); alcohol; tobacco; poor diet; stress; obesity and lack of physical activity. Having several risk factors does NOT mean that one will get cancer. Conversely, absence of risk factors does not mean that one will not get cancer.

The suggestions and information presented in this book are primarily focused on <u>prevention</u> of various cancer types through avoidance of the known risk factors for the specific cancer type. When known, information about food items or actions that could shrink or slow down growth of tumors is included. It is important to note that, there is no definitive cure, treatment or preventive measure that is known and certain for any specific type of cancer at this time.

Few words on phytochemicals, antioxidants, free radicals ...

Phytochemicals are substances or compounds found in many plants. They are also known by other names among them antioxidants and flavonoids. While thousands of phytochemicals have been discovered, very few have been studied in detail. Some of the better known phytochemicals (antioxidants) are beta carotene, Vitamin C, folic acid and Vitamin E.

Various studies and many experts suggest that the risk of cancer can be significantly reduced by eating more fruits, vegetables, beans and whole grains that contain phytochemicals. There is some evidence that certain phytochemicals may prevent formation of tumors, or suppress cancer development. But there is no data that supports taking phytochemical supplements is as effective as consuming fruits, vegetables, beans and grains as part of a normal diet. Nor are supplements regulated by the FDA. Thus, taking phytochemicals in form of supplements is not recommended.

One group of these compounds, known as antioxidants, may protect our cells against free radicals. Free radicals are molecules produced by our body as it breaks down food or by exposure to things such as tobacco smoke or radiation. Free radicals can damage our cell's DNA and are linked to certain diseases including cancer. Antioxidants are thought to eliminate free radicals, and slow down oxidation, which is a natural process that leads to damage to the cells and tissue in our body.

Another group of these compounds is known as flavonoids. Some studies suggest that some of these compounds may protect against hormone-dependent cancers such as breast and prostate cancers. Another group of flavonoids act as antioxidants, and thus have protective and anti-cancer properties.

A third group of Phytochemicals, called Allyl Sulfides, may help our body get rid of harmful chemicals and strengthen our immune system.

Many of the dietary recommendations that you find in this book are based on the various known phytochemical content and their effect on various types of cancer.

General Considerations for Defeating Cancer

Despite all the advances made in cancer research over the last several decades, per 2012 estimates from American Cancer Society (ACS), one third of Americans diagnosed with cancer die within the first five years. Considering there is over 1.6 million new cases of cancer per annum (2012 ACS estimate), this translates to an unacceptably high number of fatalities, and is a clear indication of inadequacy of existing capabilities to prevent and treat this terrible disease. In a nutshell, the prevailing cancer treatment is based on either surgery to remove affected tissue and organs, or destruction of our body cells through chemotherapy and radiation with the hope that the cancer cells will also get killed in the process. There are newer treatment paradigms emerging (e.g., cancer vaccines and adoptive immunotherapy which are the personalized medicine approaches to cancer treatment) but they are just that, too new and emerging. There has been very limited curative treatments to-date, and only in clinical trials.

Much too often patients die from the cancer treatment and not the cancer. Much too often patients refuse treatment due to unacceptable side effects, unacceptable risk-reward ratio, or because they are too weak to receive further treatment.

On the other hand, per ACS estimate, environmental factors (i.e., factors that we can control) account for 75-80% of cancer cases and deaths in the US. We need to recognize these factors and take appropriate action to avoid them and reduce our risk of getting cancer.

A common criticism of the conventional approach to cancer is that diet, free-radicals, toxins and other environmental factors are neglected. Medical community and the Pharmaceutical industry are focused on eliminating cancer cells, not cancer-causing factors. As a result, for the foreseeable future, we must take it upon ourselves to take actions to reduce our risk of getting cancer. And until there is further progress in conventional approach to cancer treatment, cancer patients and the health care community must actively seek and further explore various alternative and complementary medicine (ACM) and therapies available to them. A number of western European countries and China have successfully integrated ACM into the conventional approach to prevention and treatment of cancer.

While the focus of this book is on nutrition, we will also mention various herbal remedies and complementary therapies that are available to you. It is beyond the scope of this book, to discuss all these options in detail. But we highly encourage you to learn about these ACMs and discuss them with your natural health care provider.

To combat cancer we must recognize the main factors identified as culprits and develop an action plan to deal with each. The factors most often mentioned include: nutritional deficiencies, environmental toxins, stress, smoking, free radicals, and excess weight. Recent studies have also found a link between inflammation (our immune system natural reaction to injuries, allergies, germs and the like) and cancer.

For dealing with environmental toxins and free radicals attributed to pollution, chemicals and smoking, there are a number of detoxification programs, multi-day fasts or cleansing diets that are explicitly designed to address this critical need. There are also a number of nutrients and foods that are considered helpful in detoxification of our body, and are mentioned separately in this book.

As for the remaining factors, the guidelines provided in this book are designed to augment a well-balanced diet with antioxidants or cancer fighting foods, boost your immune system, and minimize or eliminate the damage from free radicals that are created through your food intake. Separate guidelines are also provided for dealing with obesity and stress.

One nutrition-centric approach that has been controversial but worthy of further investigation is a diet that is focused on increasing the alkalinity (or reducing the acidity) of our body tissue. There are a number of studies that suggest that the cancer cells are less likely to survive an alkaline tissue environment. A separate chapter on alkaline diet is included in this book.

There are a number of factors that are considered by some as culprits in causing cancer. While there are some books and reports published on these factors, there remains some skepticism and controversy about accuracy of such claims. But for the sake of completeness, we are including this list of suspects for your information: prescription and non-prescription drugs (due to chemical toxins), micro-waved foods, fast foods, various soda (since they can block absorption of certain nutrients), high fructose syrups, non-stick cookware, farmed fish and non-organic meat and poultry (due to growth hormones, antibiotics and chemicals fed to these animals), pork, shellfish, skin care lotions including sun-block creams, deodorants, air fresheners, all man-made and processed foods, swimming pools & steam rooms (due to chlorine), and fluorescent lighting.

In closing, remember that it is your body and it is your life. Your best ally is a strong immune system. Take actions to boost it. Remain skeptical of anyone who promises a miracle cure. And remain just as skeptical of anyone who dismisses other approaches too quickly in favor of their own. No single organization, clinic, or expert has the monopoly on the truth when it comes to cancer. And considering that cancer represents a several hundred billion dollars per year business in the US, far too many experts and organizations have a conflict of interest in their position on how to deal with cancer.

Choose these for Cancer Risk & HT

Top 5 items to consume:

Cod Liver Fish Oil; Garlic; Fish (wild fish);
Artichoke, Mushrooms & Peppers; Shellfish; &
Exercise;

Food items & actions that could improve your health or reduce your risk (within a food group, most helpful items are listed first):

Meat, Fish & Poultry

Salmon (pink); **Sturgeon**; **White fish**; **Herring**; Trout; Spot; **Tuna (blue fin)**; **Oysters**; **Smelt**; **Anchovy**; **Caviar**; **Mussels**; **Wolffish**; **Pompano fish**; **Mackerel**; **Whiting**; **Crab (Dungeness)**; Cisco (smoked); Pollock; Mullet; Marlin; Swordfish; Sucker; Bass (freshwater); Drum; Sablefish; Shad; Bluefish; Lobster (spiny); Tilapia; Crab (Alaskan King); Yellowtail; Halibut; Conch; Surimi; Cisco; Catfish; Walleye; Bass (striped); Tilefish; Crab (snow); Lingcod; Octopus; Bass (seabass); Mackerel (king); Clams; Scup; Cusk; Fish roe; Milkfish; Snapper; Snail; Crab (Blue); Burbot; Butterfish; Flatfish (flounder & sole); Ling; Tuna (yellowfin); Pout; Eel; Crayfish; Haddock; Northern pike; Turbot; Chicken breast (no skin); Pumpkinseed sunfish; Seatrout; Rockfish; Dolphinfish (Mahi-Mahi); Salmon (smoked, Lox); Shrimp; Cuttlefish; **Avoid heavy metal loaded fish;**

Eggs, Beans, Nuts and Seeds

Peas (sugar/snap); **Peas (green)**; **Soybeans (dried)**; Beans (yardlong); Lentils; Peas (split); Beans: adzuki, black, mung, navy, pinto; Pigeon peas; Other Beans; Black-eyed peas; Seeds (flaxseed)[1]; Alfalfa sprouts; Soybeans (green); Seeds (chia); Chickpeas; Seeds (breadnut tree); Lupin; Egg substitute; Ginkgo nuts;

Fruits & Juices (Five servings of fruits & vegetables daily)

Avoid non-organic. Avoid sugared juices or from concentrate; Wash fruits & vegetables well and peel their skin; Blackberries; Cranberries; Lemon; Raspberries; Rhubarb; Gooseberries; Acerola; Olives; Apricots; Boysenberries; Cantaloupe; Currants (raw); Grapefruit; Guava; Oranges; Papaya; Peaches; Plum; Watermelon; Other Berries; Orange juice; Pumelo (Shaddock); Pitanga; Passion fruit; Kiwi fruit; Mango; Persimmons; Lime; Kumquats; Abiyuch; Nectarine; Natal Plum (Carissa); Starfruit; Apricots (dried); Pomegranate; Rowal; Blueberries; Cranberry juice; Jujube (fruit); Tangerines; Grapefruit juice; Pineapple; Plantains; Durian; Breadfruit; Apples; Peaches (dried); Litchi; Dried Fruits; Longans; Pineapple juice; Tamarind; Pears; Apple juice; Grapes; Honeydew melon; Cherries; Figs; Banana; Quince; Grape juice; Strawberries; Pomegranate juice; Raisins; Dates; Prune juice; Avocado;

Vegetables (Five servings of fruits & vegetables daily)

Avoid non-organic. Wash fruits & vegetables well and peel their skin; Garlic (use raw or crushed but not heated immediately); Artichoke; Winged beans leaves; Mushrooms (Chanterelle); Peppers (jalapeno); Peppers (pimento); Mushrooms (shitake); Cloud ear fungus; Chicory greens; Taro leaves; Tomatoes (sun-dried); Mushrooms (portabella); Peppers (hot chili); Broccoli; Cauliflower; Endive; Arrowroot; Onions (2-5 oz. of fresh onion daily, or 1 tsp. onion juice 3-4 times a day); Amaranth leaves; Arugula; Balsam pear leafy tips; Beet greens; Bell peppers; Bok choy; Borage; Broccoli (Chinese); Brussels sprouts; Various Cabbage; Celtuce; Chrysanthemum (Garland); Chrysanthemum Leaves; Collards; Cowpeas leafy tips; Dandelion Greens; Epazote; Garden cress; Green beans; Green onions (scallions); Kale; Kohlrabi; Lambsquarters; Various Lettuce; Mustard greens; Mustard spinach; Okra; Peppers; Pokeberry shoots; Pumpkin; Pumpkin flowers; Purslane; Radishes; Rutabaga; Sesbania Flower; Spinach; Squash: Butternut, Hubbard; Sweet potatoes leaves; Swiss chard; Taro (Tahitian); Tomato juice; Tomatoes; Turnip greens; Vine spinach (Basella); Watercress; Zucchini; Other Vegetables;

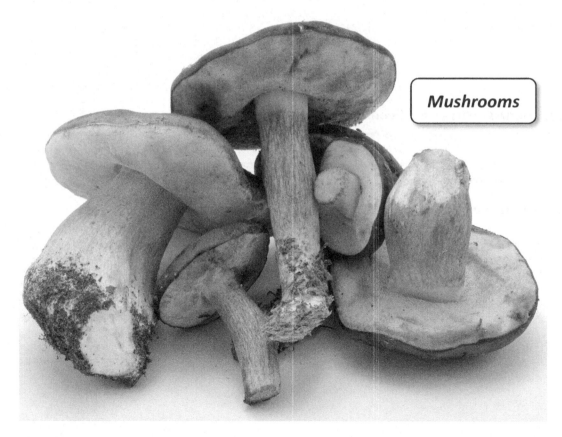

Mushrooms

Breads, Grains, Cereals, Pasta

Corn bran; Barley; Buckwheat; Oats; Triticale; Rye grain; Sorghum grain; Corn; Quinoa; Rice cakes (Brown rice); Rice (wild); Millet; Rice (brown);

Dairy Products, Fats & Oils

Fish oil (cod liver); **Fish oil (sardine)**; **Fish oil (salmon)**; **Other Fish oil**; Yogurt; Oil (flaxseed);

Desserts, Snacks, Beverages

Tea (green; do not brew or drink boiling hot); Water (clean water, not tap water); Wine (red); Tea (plain);

Herbs & Spices, Fast Foods, Prepared Foods

Coriander/Cilantro; Parsley; Soup (minestrone); Thyme (fresh); Soup (vegetable); Cayenne (red) pepper; Ginger; Corn salad; Miso; Tomato paste; Tempeh; Mints; Kimchi; Spearmint (fresh); Peppermint; Tofu; Dill weed; Sauerkraut; Cinnamon; Fish stock; Basil (fresh); Mace; Nutmeg; Rosemary (fresh); Turmeric; Soup (tomato); Pepper (black); Succotash; Balsamic vinegar; Vinegar; Soup (clam chowder);

Alternative Therapies & Miscellaneous

Wild fish and free range animals (avoid animals raised on antibiotics or grains); **Consult your doctor (ask for cancer screening tests)**; **Exercise (Cardiovascular, weight training, jogging, walking, or cycling)**; Anti-inflammation diet; Organic cold-pressed oils; Organically grown foods; Fresh (uncooked) fruits/veg's;

Key Nutrients & Herbal Meds

Omega-3 fatty acids (breast, prostate and colon cancers in particular**)**; Goji berry; Beta Carotene (do not take in supplement form); Bugleweed; Fiber; Foxglove; Psyllium; Vitamin B-3 (Niacin; in nicotinic acid form, not recommended as supplement or drug);

Do not choose these for Cancer Risk & HT

Top 5 items to avoid:

Sweets; Luncheon (Processed) Meats; Fast Foods; Shortening; Salad Dressings;

Avoid or consume much less of the following (within a food group, most harmful items are listed first):

Meat, Fish & Poultry

Bacon; Beef (cured brkfst strips); Beef jerky sticks; Beef tongue; Salami; Bologna; Chorizo; Frankfurters; Luncheon meats; Pepperoni; Pork breakfast strips; Pork headcheese; Pork skins; Pork spare ribs; Sausages; Turkey skins; Pork ribs; Lamb tongue; Pork liver cheese; Pastrami; Lamb ribs; Beef (ground); Lamb brain; Chicken skin; Beef chuck/brisket; Organ meats; Pork shoulder; Corned beef; Beef ribs; Cured Meats; Goose; Pork; Lamb; Bear meat; Chicken wings; Beef; Beaver meat; Chicken dark meat; Croaker; Squab (pigeon); Meat (limit consumption of red meat; choose organic); Quail; Frog legs; Bison/buffalo meat; Shark; Rabbit meat; Goat meat; Boar meat; Venison; Veal shoulder; Tuna (canned); Caribou meat; Veal loin; Pheasant; Duck (no skin); Beef filet mignon; Orange roughy; Veal shank; Turkey giblets; Guinea hen; Abalone; Turkey dark meat; White fish (smoked);

Instead _Choose_: Chicken liver; Squid (Calamari); Sheepshead; Sardines; Pheasant breast; Lobster; Quail breast; Carp; Scallops; Perch; Turkey breast; Whelk; Cod; Grouper; Monkfish;

Eggs, Beans, Nuts and Seeds

Pili nuts; Butternuts; Pine nuts; Seeds (pumpkin/squash); Hickory nuts; Seeds (watermelon); Walnuts (black); Cashew nuts; Seeds: cottonseed, sesame; Pistachio nuts; Seeds (safflower); Pecans; Brazil nuts; Beechnuts; Peanuts; Almonds; Egg yolk; Hazelnuts or Filberts; Acorns; Coconut meat (dried); Coconut meat (raw); Egg (hard-boiled); Seeds (sunflower); Egg (raw); Cornnuts; Coconut milk; Egg (duck); Macadamia nuts;

Instead _Choose_: Breadfruit seeds; Egg white; Walnuts; Chestnuts;

Fruits & Juices

Avoid sugared or made from concentrate juices. There are no fruits that could worsen your conditions.

Vegetables

Fiddlehead ferns (some varieties are carcinogenic);

Breads, Grains, Cereals, Pasta

Danish pastry; Donuts; Granola bars; Muffins (blueberry); Muffins (wheat bran); Sweet rolls; Crackers (wheat); Croissant; Biscuits; Cereal (granola); Muffins (oat bran); Cereals; Crackers (milk); Bread (cornbread); Wheat germ; Bread (banana); Bread sticks; Waffles; Muffins (corn); Crackers (saltines); Crackers (whole-wheat); Rolls (Kaiser); Bagels; Rolls (hamburger/hot dog); Noodles (Chinese chow Mein); English muffins; Rolls (whole-wheat dinner); Melba toast; Cereal (wheat germ); Cereal (rice crisps); Rolls (French); Wheat; Bread (white); Cereal (shredded wheat); Rice (white); Whole-wheat; Crackers (matzo); Toasted bread; Cereal (cream of wheat); Wheat bran; Semolina; Cereal (raisin bran); Bread (Italian); Cereal (whole-wheat); Spaghetti; Cereal (corn flakes); Bread (pumpernickel); Cereal (bran flakes); Couscous; Tortillas (corn); Bread (oat bran); Bread (wheat germ); Bread (French/Sourdough); Noodles (egg); Spelt; Spaghetti (whole-wheat); Pasta; Noodles (Japanese); Noodles (rice); Bulgur; Oatmeal (cereal); Bread (whole-wheat); English muffins (whole wheat)

Instead ***Choose:*** *Spaghetti (spinach); Amaranth; Cornmeal (whole-grain); Oat bran; Durum wheat; Rice bran; English muffins (whole-wheat); Bread (whole-wheat); Oatmeal (cereal);*

Dairy Products, Fats & Oils

Cheese (American); Non-dairy creamers; Vegetable shortening; Cheese (Romano); Oil (wheat germ); Butter (salted); Cheese spread; Cheese (Parmesan); Hydrogenated vegetable oil; Butter (unsalted); Oil (sesame); Oil (tomato seeds); Cheese: Pimento, Feta, Blue; Oil (walnut); Other Cheese; Fat (chicken, turkey); Other Oils; Fat (duck); Lard; Cream (whipped); Margarine; Margarine-like spreads; Milk (chocolate); Milk (whole); Fat (beef/lamb/pork); Milk (skim); Oil (canola); Oil (hazelnut); Cheese (Gjetost); Cheese (Ricotta); Milk (1% fat); Milk (2% fat); Sour cream; Buttermilk; Cream; Cheese (Cottage);

Instead ***Choose:*** *Oil (olive); Whey (sweet);*

Desserts, Snacks, Beverages

Brownies; Cakes; Candies (peanut bar); Cookies; Cream puffs/Éclair; Pie (fried, fruit); Pie crust; Puff pastry; Tortilla chips; Halvah (candy); Coffeecake; Pie (pecan); Ice cream cones; Pies; Cheesecake; Peanut butter; Candies (peanut brittle); Dessert toppings; Fruit leather/rolls; Candies; Potato chips; Coffee liqueur; Frostings; Taro chips; After-dinner mints; Chocolate mousse; Potato sticks; Crème de menthe; Ice cream (chocolate); Marshmallows; Honey; Chewing gum; Ice cream (vanilla); Frozen yogurt; Pretzels; Popcorn (oil popped); Carob (candy); Pancakes; Sherbet; Candies (hard); Jams & Preserves; Jellies; Chocolate (sweet); Molasses; Soft (carbonated) drinks; Milk shakes; Eggnog; Applesauce; Piña colada; Pie (pumpkin); Hot chocolate; Ginger ale; Tonic water; Lemonade; 80+ proof distilled alc. bev.; Fruit punch; Sports drinks; Chocolate (dark); Whiskey; Red Bull (drink); Malted drinks (nonalcoholic); Popcorn (air popped); Coffee;

Instead ***choose:*** *Coffee (decaf); Tea (herbal); Soy milk; Beer; Wine (white);*

Herbs & Spices, Fast Foods, Prepared Foods

Breaded shrimp; Cheeseburger; Hush puppies; Nachos; Onion rings; Pizza; Salad dressings; Hot dog; Sausage (meatless); Hamburger; Taco shells; Sugar (table, powder); Chicken Nuggets; Hash brown potatoes; Potato salad; French toast; Tahini; Barbecue sauce; Foie gras or liver pate; Potato pancakes; Syrups; Hummus; Mayonnaise; French fries; Sauce (Hoisin); Sugar (brown); Teriyaki sauce; Sauces; Soup (beef barley); Ketchup; Syrup (malt); Cottonseed meal; Macaroni; Natto; Soy sauce; Tabasco sauce; Beef broth; Corn cakes; Pickle (sweet); Beef stock; Tofu (fried); Croutons; Salt (table); Soup (chicken noodle); Poppy seed; Falafel; Egg rolls (veg); Chicken broth; Pickle relish;

Instead Choose: Cocoa; Chervil; Horseradish; Marjoram; Sage; Tarragon; Soup (veg/beef); Cardamom; Chives; Cloves; Oregano; Saffron; Cornmeal (whole-grain); Fennel seeds; Pickle (cucumber); Gravies (canned); Mustard seed; Capers; Mustard; Cole slaw; Sugar (maple);

Alternative Therapies & Miscellaneous

Smoking/Tobacco; Deep-fried foods; 2+ alcoholic drinks/day; Cheese made w/whole milk; Excess body weight; Pesticide-loaded crops (avoid non-organic foods. if not possible, wash fruits/vegs well and peel off their skin); Processed or Refined foods (avoid any and all manufactured foods); Aspartame (Equal, check low fat/diet products for this additive); Corn syrup; Air pollutants; Food additives Nitrates/Nitrites; Smoked fish/foods; Harsh chemicals & fumes; Non-organic foods (due to heavy use of pesticide/hormones in farmed plants/animals); Radiation (from x-rays, television, microwave, computer, cell phones); Stress; Canned foods;

Key Nutrients & Herbal Meds

Trans fatty acids; Omega-6 fatty acid (LA); Fat (saturated); Betel Nut; Mercury & other heavy metals (found in deep sea fish); Sugar (refined); Alcohol;

Stress (& HT)

Everyone experiences some sort of stress almost every day. Stress is our brain's response to a demand. Not everyone reacts to the same events or demands the same way. What may be stressful to one person may not be to another. It is stress that drives us to act, and in some cases such as survival situations, perform beyond our normal abilities. However, long term or chronic stress can lead to a variety of problems including illnesses such as high blood pressure, depression and cancer.

Chronic stress can be caused by a number of factors, among them: bad childhood experiences (whose pain and impact you have never been able to escape), poverty and helplessness, an unhappy marriage, never-ending tension and violence all around you, a wrong job or career, and a dysfunctional family.

Chronic stress challenges our mind and body over a long time, and thus may require an on-going treatment over an extended period of time.

Choose these for Stress & HT

Top 5 items to consume:

Fish; Garlic & Ginger; Cod Liver Fish Oil; Shellfish; & Exercise;

Food items and actions that could improve your health (within a food group, most helpful items are listed first):

Meat, Fish & Poultry

Anchovy; Bluefish; Cisco (smoked); Mackerel; Mackerel (king); Marlin; Salmon (pink); Spot; Sturgeon; Swordfish; Trout; Tuna (blue fin); White fish; Herring; Sablefish; Tilefish; Bass (striped); Smelt; Tuna (yellowfin); Halibut; Bass (seabass); Wolffish; Pollock; Salmon (smoked, Lox); Sucker; Caviar; Mullet; Bass (freshwater); Drum; Whiting; Shad; Mussels; Milkfish; Cisco; Oysters; Surimi; Pompano fish; Tilapia; Seatrout; Walleye; Yellowtail; Lobster (spiny); Octopus; Crab (Dungeness); White fish (smoked); Dolphinfish (Mahi-Mahi); Snapper; Flatfish (flounder & sole); Butterfish; Scup; Catfish; Lingcod; Clams; Rockfish; Cusk; Burbot; Carp; Perch; Haddock; Grouper; Crab (Alaskan King); Northern pike; Sheepshead; Chicken breast (no skin); Pumpkinseed sunfish; Crab (snow); Conch; Ling; Snail; Beef filet mignon; Fish roe; Sardines; Turbot; Cuttlefish; Monkfish; Veal loin; Cod; Pout; Whelk; Caribou meat; Veal shank; Crab (Blue); Eel; Lobster; Shrimp; Beef rib eye; Shark; Scallops; Pheasant breast; Orange roughy; Beef top sirloin; Veal shoulder; Rabbit meat; Crayfish; Beef round steak; Beef tenderloin/T-bone/porterhouse; Tuna (canned); Squid (Calamari); Quail breast; Chicken liver; Lamb leg; Pork loin/sirloin; Turkey dark meat; Pheasant; Bison/buffalo meat; Turkey breast; Venison; Goat meat; Turkey liver; Boar meat; Liver; Beaver meat; Abalone; Croaker; Beef shank;

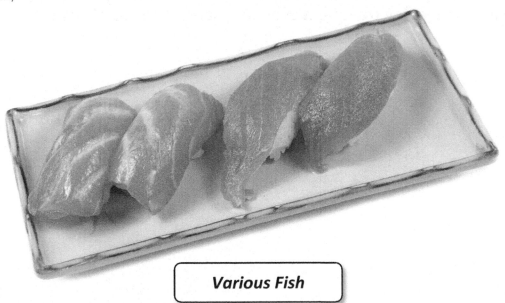

Various Fish

Eggs, Beans, Nuts and Seeds

Peas (sugar/snap); Peas (green); Soybeans (dried); Seeds: chia, flaxseed; Beans (yardlong); Seeds (breadnut tree); Beans: yellow, hyacinth; Lentils; Egg white; Beans: moth beans, fava; Black-eyed peas; Alfalfa sprouts; Egg substitute; Beans: mung, pinto, great northern; Peas (split); Egg (duck); Pigeon peas;

Fruits & Juices

Acerola; Lemon; Orange juice; Pumelo (Shaddock); Guava; Jujube (fruit); Papaya; Strawberries; Persimmons; Abiyuch; Kumquats; Pineapple; Currants (raw); Natal Plum (Carissa); Grapefruit juice; Oranges; Passion fruit; Longans; Cantaloupe; Raisins; Litchi; Litchi (dried); Banana; Lime; Starfruit; Kiwi fruit; Prune juice; Apple juice; Durian; Olives; Breadfruit; Berries; Peaches; Pitanga; Nectarine; Plum; Watermelon; Tamarind; Grapefruit; Mango; Banana (dried); Pomegranate juice; Pomegranate; Rowal; Plantains; Pears; Dried Fruits; Cherries; Dates; Grapes; Grape juice; Apples; Apricots; Honeydew melon; Pineapple juice; **Avoid sugared and made from concentrate juices;**

Vegetables

Garlic; **Winged beans leaves**; **Peppers (jalapeno)**; **Peppers (pimento)**; **Taro leaves**; **Peppers (hot chili)**; **Broccoli**; **Cauliflower**; Amaranth leaves; Balsam pear; Balsam pear leafy tips; Bell peppers (red); Bok choy; Brussels sprouts; Cabbage (red); Garden cress; Kohlrabi; Lambsquarters; Mustard spinach; Peppers; Pokeberry shoots; Sesbania Flower; Taro (Tahitian); Vine spinach (Basella); Grape leaves; Cowpeas leafy tips; Mustard greens; Bell peppers (green); Borage; Epazote; Cabbage (green); Watercress; Kale; Broccoli (Chinese); Cabbage (savoy); Turnip greens; Mushrooms: Chanterelle, shitake, Cloud ear fungus; Yam; Onions; Artichoke; Pumpkin flowers; Dandelion Greens; Mushrooms (portabella); Purslane; Kelp; Lotus root; Arrowroot; Arrowhead; Chicory greens; Mushrooms (Morel); Collards; Arugula; Squash (Acorn); Sweet potatoes leaves; Tomatoes (sun-dried); Fiddlehead ferns; Spinach; Shallots; Chrysanthemum (Garland); Chrysanthemum Leaves; Rutabaga; Green onions (scallions); Nopal; Taro; Radishes; Cucumber with peel; Turnips; Celtuce; Mushrooms (Jew's ear); Beet greens; Potatoes w/skin;

Breads, Grains, Cereals, Pasta

Rice bran; Cereals: corn flakes, rice crisps; Rice cakes (Brown rice); English muffins (whole-wheat); Cereals: raisin bran, bran flakes; Wheat bran; Triticale; Cereal (shredded wheat); Quinoa; Corn bran; Bread (whole-wheat); Millet; Rice (wild); Spaghetti (spinach); Sorghum grain;

Dairy Products, Fats & Oils

Fish oil (cod liver); **Fish oil (sardine)**; **Fish oil (salmon)**; **Other Fish oil**; Oil (flaxseed); Oil (olive); Yogurt;

Desserts, Snacks, Beverages

Red Bull (drink); Tea (green, decaffeinated in particular); Water; Coffee (decaf);

Herbs & Spices, Fast Foods, Prepared Foods

Ginger; Corn salad; Thyme (fresh); Fish stock; Soup (clam chowder); Kimchi; Cottonseed meal; Cayenne (red) pepper; Cinnamon; Tofu; Succotash; Parsley; Dill weed; Cornmeal (whole-grain); Sauerkraut;

Alternative Therapies & Miscellaneous

Consult your doctor (determine if you suffer from adrenal fatigue); **Exercise (Including Cardiovascular, Weight Training, Walking, Jogging, or Cycling);** Wild fish and free range animals; Fresh (uncooked) fruits/veg's; Laugh, laughter; Meditation; Organically grown foods; Sleep 6-8 hours regularly; Take a vacation!; Yoga;

Key Nutrients & Herbal Meds

Omega-3 fatty acids; **Vitamin C**; Ashwaganda (root & leaf); Calcium; Ginseng (Asian); Ginseng (Siberian); Licorice (root); Magnesium; Vitamin B-3 (Niacin; in nicotinic acid form, not recommended as supplement or drug); Vitamin B-6 (Pyridoxine); Vitamin D;

Do not choose these for Stress & HT

Top 5 items to avoid:

Chocolate & Sweets; Salad Dressings; Nuts; Luncheon Meats; Margarine & Hydrogenated Vegetable Oil;

Avoid or consume much less of the following (within a food group, most harmful items are listed first):

Meat, Fish & Poultry

Sausages; Luncheon meats; Frankfurters; Pepperoni; Salami; Pork skins; Pastrami; Chicken skin; Chorizo; Beef jerky sticks; Pork liver cheese; Bologna; Pork breakfast strips; Pork headcheese; Beef (cured brkfst strips); Bacon; Turkey skins; Goose; Corned beef; Organ Meats; Cured Meats; Chicken wings; Pork ribs; Pork spare ribs; Lamb ribs; Pork; Chicken dark meat; Beef chuck/brisket; Squab (pigeon); Quail; Frog legs; Beef ribs; Duck (no skin);

Instead <u>choose</u>: Guinea hen; Veal liver; Bear meat; Lamb liver; Beef (ground); Pork leg/ham; Lamb;

Eggs, Beans, Nuts and Seeds

Hickory nuts; Butternuts; Pili nuts; Beechnuts; Pine nuts; Pecans; Peanuts; Pistachio nuts; Acorns; Walnuts (black); Walnuts; Brazil nuts; Cashew nuts; Coconut meat (dried); Coconut meat (raw); Seeds (sesame); Cornnuts; Seeds: pumpkin/squash, watermelon, safflower, cottonseed; Almonds; Hazelnuts or Filberts; Chestnuts; Soy milk; Breadfruit seeds; Macadamia nuts; Ginkgo nuts; Coconut milk; Beans (black); Soybeans (green); Chickpeas; Seeds (sunflower); Beans: navy, baked, adzuki; Egg (hard-boiled); Egg (raw); Lupin;

Instead <u>Choose</u>: Beans: lima, winged, kidney; Egg yolk;

Fruit & Juices

Gooseberries; Figs; Figs (dried); Rhubarb; Apricots (dried); Longans (dried); Cranberry juice; **Avoid sugared or made from concentrate juices;**

Instead <u>Choose</u>: Prunes (dried); Blueberries; Tangerines; Avocado; Loganberry; Quince; Cranberries;

Vegetables

Leeks; Beets; Endive; Celery; Green beans; Squash (Spaghetti); Tomatoes; Parsnips; Eggplant; Sweet potatoes; Pumpkin;

Instead <u>Choose</u>: Potato; Fennel (Bulb); Swiss chard; Hearts of palm; Okra; Squash (Butternut); Carrots; Cabbage (Cruciferous) family; Lettuce (head); Lettuce (loose leaf); Lettuce (Romaine); Wasabi root; Tomato juice; Squash (Hubbard); Zucchini; Artichoke (Jerusalem); Asparagus;

Breads, Grains, Cereals, Pasta

Sweet rolls; Danish pastry; Crackers (wheat); Donuts; Croissant; Granola bars; Muffins (blueberry); Crackers (milk); Bread sticks; Bread (banana); Cereal (granola); Crackers (whole-wheat); Rolls (Kaiser); Biscuits; Crackers (saltines); Muffins (corn); Melba toast; Muffins (wheat bran); Bread (cornbread); Waffles; Noodles (Chinese chow Mein); Cereal (cream of wheat); Wheat germ; Rolls (whole-wheat dinner); Rolls (hamburger/hot dog); Crackers (matzo); Rolls (French); Muffins (oat bran); Noodles (egg); Bread (Italian); Amaranth; Bread (pumpernickel); Wheat; Bread (oat bran); Couscous; Bagels; Bread (white); Pasta; English muffins; Tortillas (corn); Bread (French/Sourdough); Spaghetti (whole-wheat); Barley; Noodles (rice); Whole-wheat; Spaghetti; Buckwheat;

Instead choose: Oats; Oatmeal (cereal); Rye grain; Spelt; Popcorn (air popped); Oat bran; Cereal (whole-wheat); Cereal (wheat germ); Semolina; Rice (brown); Rice (white); Noodles (Japanese); Bread (wheat germ); Durum wheat; Toasted bread; Corn; Bulgur;

Dairy Products, Fats & Oils

Non-dairy creamers; Margarine; Hydrogenated vegetable oil; Margarine-like spreads; Oils: sesame, tomato seeds, walnut; Fat (chicken, turkey, duck); Oil (tea seed); Vegetable shortening; Oil (corn); Oil (poppy seed); Lard; Other Oils; Butter; Cheese (Cream); Cheese (Goat); Milk (chocolate); Cream (whipped); Cheese (Brie); Fat (beef/lamb/pork); Cheese (Ricotta); Cheese spread; Various cheese; Milk (whole); Sour cream; Cheese (Gjetost); Cheese (Gruyere); Milk (skim); Cheese (Swiss); Milk (1% fat); Buttermilk; Milk (2% fat); Whey (sweet);

Instead choose: Cheese (Cottage); Cream;

Desserts, Snacks, Beverages

Cake (chocolate); Puff pastry; Cookies (chocolate chip); Brownies; Ice cream (chocolate); Coffeecake; Cake (yellow); Cheesecake; Chocolate; Pie (fried, fruit); Chocolate mousse; Cream puffs/Éclair; Cake (pound); Candies (peanut brittle); Coffee liqueur; Cookies; Chocolate (dark); Pudding; Cakes; Ice cream cones; Pie (apple); Pie crust; Frostings; Pies; Crème de menthe; Chocolate (sweet); Dessert toppings; After-dinner mints; Chewing gum; Sherbet; Jams & Preserves; Candies (caramel); Ice cream (vanilla); Candies (hard); Marshmallows; Honey; Peanut butter; Candies (peanut bar); Jellies; Taro chips; Piña colada; Frozen yogurt; Popcorn (oil popped); Hot chocolate; Pretzels; Carob (candy); Halvah (candy); Tortilla chips; 80+ proof distilled alc. bev.; Whiskey; Fruit punch; Applesauce; Milk shakes; Eggnog; Pancakes; Lemonade; Ginger ale; Potato chips; Soft (carbonated) drinks; Wine (red); Wine (white); Beer; Malted drinks (nonalcoholic); Fruit leather/rolls; Sports drinks; Tonic water; Potato sticks; Tea (plain);

Instead choose: Molasses; Popcorn (air popped); Candies (sesame crunch); Tea (herbal); Coffee;

Herbs & Spices, Fast Foods, Prepared Foods

Salad dressings; **Potato salad**; **Teriyaki sauce**; **Hot dog**; **Soy sauce**; **Syrup (chocolate)**; **Onion rings**; **Pizza**; **Tahini**; **French fries**; **Breaded shrimp**; **Sugar (table, powder)**; **Mayonnaise**; **French toast**; **Hash brown potatoes**; **Foie gras or liver pate**; **Syrup (maple)**; **Syrup (table blends)**; **Hush puppies**; Chicken Nuggets; Nachos; Cheeseburger; Hamburger; Sausage (meatless); Barbecue sauce; Egg rolls (veg); Hummus; Tofu (fried); Sugar (brown); Sauce (Hoisin); Taco shells; Ketchup; Macaroni; Poppy seed; Natto; Sauces; Soup (beef barley); Cocoa; Miso; Pickle (sweet); Croutons; Potato pancakes; Soup (vegetable); Sugar (maple); Soup (minestrone); Tomato paste; Turmeric; Syrup (sorghum); Soup (tomato); Salt (table); Corn cakes; Cloves; Oregano;

Instead <u>choose</u>: Mints; Rosemary (fresh); Pickle (cucumber); Pickle relish; Balsamic vinegar; Herbs & Spices; Gravies; Horseradish; Vinegar; Cole slaw; Mustard; Syrup (malt); Capers; Tempeh; Falafel; Soup (chicken noodle); Soup (veg/beef);

Alternative Therapies & Miscellaneous

Deep-fried foods; **Cheese made w/whole milk**; Smoking/Tobacco; Corn syrup; 2+ alcoholic drinks/day; Excess body weight; Birth control pills; Processed or Refined foods; Stress; FD&C yellow dye #5. Tartrazine; Artificial sweeteners; Baking using butter;

Key Nutrients & Herbal Meds

Omega-6 fatty acid (LA); **Trans fatty acids**; Fat (saturated); Oxalate; Alcohol; Sugar (refined);

Vitamin D Deficiency (& HT)

Vitamin D Deficiency is a common problem for many people especially the older people. Vitamin D is a critical nutrient for your body in particular for stronger bones, muscle movements, nerve function and immune system well-being.

You will develop this deficiency if you don't absorb enough Vitamin D from your diet, you don't get enough exposure to the sun (especially during the winter months), your skin cannot convert the sun exposure to Vitamin D (as in elderly and darker skin), or you are obese. You can also develop this deficiency if your body cannot properly process fats due to Celiac or Crohn's disease, since fats are required for Vitamin D absorption into your blood. Health issues with kidney and liver can also result in this deficiency because they can prevent your body to process Vitamin D.

Adults, ages 19 to 70, require 600 IU (International Units) of Vitamin D per day. Adults, ages 71 and above, require 800 IU per day.

Meeting your Vitamin D needs entirely through sun exposure or tanning is not recommended due to the risk of skin cancer. Too much Vitamin D in your blood (almost always caused by supplements) can also be harmful.

Choose these for Vitamin D Deficiency & HT

Top 5 items to consume:

Fish Oil; Fish & Shellfish; Chanterelle Mushrooms; Soybeans; Garlic & Ginger; Exercise & Get some Sun;

Food items and actions that could improve your health (within a food group, most helpful items are listed first):

Meat, Fish & Poultry

Cisco (smoked); **Mackerel**; **Marlin**; **Salmon (pink)**; **Sturgeon**; **Swordfish**; **Trout**; **White fish**; **Pompano fish**; **Tuna (blue fin)**; **Herring**; **White fish (smoked)**; **Snapper**; **Catfish**; **Carp**; **Halibut**; **Bass (seabass)**; **Shad**; **Anchovy**; Bluefish; Mackerel (king); Spot; Sablefish; Tilefish; Eel; Tuna (yellowfin); Caviar; Salmon (smoked, Lox); Mussels; Mullet; Whiting; Tilapia; Bass (striped); Smelt; Wolffish; Pollock; Sucker; Flatfish (flounder & sole); Bass (freshwater); Drum; Rockfish; Oysters; Lobster (spiny); Walleye; Perch; Crab (Dungeness); Milkfish; Yellowtail; Cisco; Crab (Alaskan King); Surimi; Sardines; Fish roe; Crab (snow); Clams; Dolphinfish (Mahi-Mahi); Seatrout; Northern pike; Octopus; Grouper; Butterfish; Scup; Lingcod; Chicken breast (no skin); Lobster; Burbot; Cusk; Haddock; Cod; Veal loin; Scallops; Pheasant breast; Ling; Monkfish; Sheepshead; Crab (Blue); Veal shank; Quail breast; Pumpkinseed sunfish; Turbot; Conch; Orange roughy; Pout; Snail;

Eggs, Beans, Nuts and Seeds

Soybeans (dried); Seeds (chia); Egg substitute; Alfalfa sprouts; Peas (sugar/snap); Peas (green);

Fruits & Juices

There are no fruits and juices that can _improve_ your conditions, but there are many that are neutral for you and are listed in the next section.

Vegetables

Mushrooms (Chanterelle); Garlic; Mushrooms (Morel); Mushrooms (shitake); Artichoke; Mushrooms (portabella); Onions; Winged beans leaves; Mushrooms (Jew's ear); Peppers (jalapeno); Peppers (pimento); Cloud ear fungus;

Breads, Grains, Cereals, Pasta

Cereal (corn flakes); Rice bran;

Dairy Products, Fats & Oils

Fish oil (cod liver); **Fish oil (sardine)**; Other Fish oil; Oil (olive); Oil (flaxseed);

Desserts, Snacks, Beverages

Tea (green);

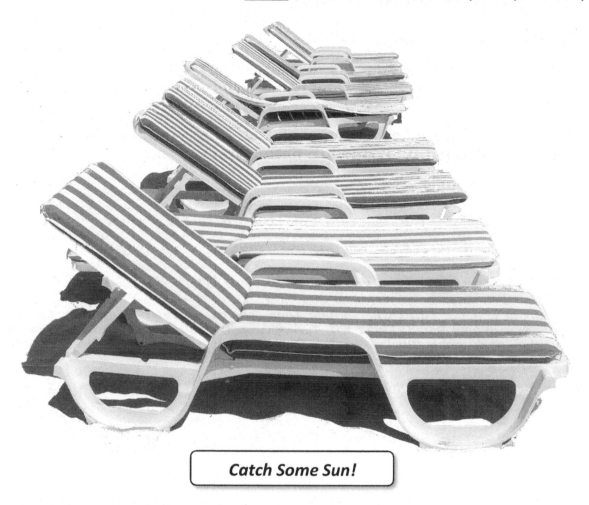

Catch Some Sun!

Herbs & Spices, Fast Foods, Prepared Foods

Ginger; Cayenne (red) pepper; Cinnamon; Fish stock; Soup (clam chowder); Miso;

Alternative Therapies & Miscellaneous

Exposure to sun (ten minutes per day); Wild fish and free range animals; Exercise;

Key Nutrients & Herbal Meds

Omega-3 fatty acids; **Vitamin D**; Vitamin B-3 (Niacin; in nicotinic acid form, not recommended as supplement or drug);

Do not choose these for Vitamin D Deficiency & HT

Top 5 items to avoid:

Chocolate; Fast Foods; Sweets; Butter & Margarine; Hydrogenated Vegetable Oil & Shortening; & Excess Body Weight;

Avoid or consume much less of the following (within a food group, most harmful items are listed first):

Meat, Fish & Poultry

Beef (cured brkfst strips); Beef jerky sticks; Salami; Bologna; Frankfurters; Luncheon meats; Pepperoni; Sausages; Pork liver cheese; Pastrami; Bacon; Pork breakfast strips; Chorizo; Corned beef; Organ Meats; Chicken skin; Pork skins; Turkey skins; Cured Meats; Goose; Lamb ribs; Beef chuck/brisket; Pork ribs/spare ribs; Chicken wings; Beef (ground); Pork; Beef ribs; Chicken dark meat; Lamb; Beaver meat; Beef; Squab (pigeon); Bear meat; Quail; Croaker; Bison/buffalo meat; Frog legs; Boar meat; Duck (no skin); Goat meat;

Instead choose: Cuttlefish; Shrimp; Tuna (canned); Beef filet mignon; Caribou meat; Crayfish; Squid (Calamari); Turkey breast; Veal shoulder; Shark; Venison; Turkey dark meat; Whelk; Guinea hen; Abalone; Pheasant; Beef rib eye; Rabbit meat;

Eggs, Beans, Nuts and Seeds

Brazil nuts; Butternuts; Hickory nuts; Pili nuts; Pine nuts; Seeds: cottonseed, pumpkin/squash, sesame, watermelon, safflower; Beechnuts; Pistachio nuts; Cashew nuts; Walnuts (black); Seeds (sunflower); Almonds; Pecans; Walnuts; Coconut meat (dried); Coconut meat (raw); Peanuts; Acorns; Egg (hard-boiled); Hazelnuts or Filberts; Egg (raw); Egg yolk; Egg (duck); Coconut milk; Chickpeas; Cornnuts; Beans (winged); Chestnuts; Beans (baked); Soybeans (green); Soy milk; Macadamia nuts;

Instead choose: Other Beans; Seeds (flaxseed); Lentils; Peas (split); Black-eyed peas; Pigeon peas; Ginkgo nuts; Egg white; Seeds (breadnut tree); Breadfruit seeds; Lupin;

Fruits & Juices

Tamarind; Avocado; Longans; Plantains; Currants (dried); Figs; Litchi; Dried Fruits; Prune juice; Grapes; Breadfruit; Cherries; Pomegranate; Quince; Rowal; Dates; Abiyuch; Kumquats; Banana; **Avoid sugared or made from concentrate fruit juices;**

Instead choose: Berries; Other fruits;

Vegetables

Peppers (ancho); Artichoke (Jerusalem); Shallots;

Instead choose: Cauliflower; Arrowroot; Chicory greens; Taro leaves; Fiddlehead ferns; Tomatoes (sun-dried); Peppers (hot chili); Broccoli; Endive; Kelp; Squash (Acorn); Potato; all other vegetables;

Breads, Grains, Cereals, Pasta

Cereal (wheat germ); Biscuits; Bread (banana); Bread (cornbread); Cereal (granola); Croissant; Danish pastry; Donuts; Granola bars; Various Muffins; Sweet rolls; Waffles; Crackers (wheat); Rolls (whole-wheat dinner); Bread sticks; Noodles (Chinese chow Mein); Crackers: milk, whole wheat, saltines; Rolls (Kaiser); Melba toast; Tortillas (corn); Wheat germ; Cereals: shredded wheat, raisin bran; Rolls (hamburger/hot dog); Bread: Italian, pumpernickel; Bagels; English muffins; Noodles (egg); Bread (white); Cereal (whole-wheat); Oatmeal (cereal); Bread: oat bran, whole-wheat; Cereal (bran flakes); Amaranth; Quinoa; Rolls (French); Spelt; Bulgur; Millet; Rice (brown); Rice (wild); Spaghetti (whole-wheat); Cereal (rice crisps); Toasted bread; English muffins (whole-wheat); Barley; Pasta;

Instead <u>choose</u>: Rice cakes (Brown rice); Wheat bran; Oats; Triticale; Rice (white); Spaghetti (spinach); Buckwheat; Croutons; Durum wheat; Oat bran; Semolina; Sorghum grain; Whole-wheat; Bread (wheat germ); Bread (French/Sourdough); Couscous; Crackers (matzo); Noodles (Japanese); Noodles (rice); Rye grain; Wheat; Cereal (cream of wheat); Corn; Spaghetti;

Dairy Products, Fats & Oils

Butter; Various Cheese; Cheese spread; Cream (whipped); Fat (chicken, duck, turkey); Hydrogenated vegetable oil; Lard; Margarine; Margarine-like spreads; Non-dairy creamers; Various Oils; Vegetable shortening; Milk (whole); Milk (chocolate); Cheese (Ricotta); Fat (beef/lamb/pork); Oils: Shea nut, canola; Sour cream; Milk (skim); Milk (1% fat); Milk (2% fat); Buttermilk; Whey (sweet); Cheese (Cottage); Cream; Yogurt;

Desserts, Snacks, Beverages

Coffee liqueur; Ice cream (chocolate); Cookies (chocolate chip); Cake (chocolate); Chocolate mousse; Sherbet; After-dinner mints; Brownies; Cakes; Candies; Cheesecake; Chewing gum; Coffeecake; Cookies; Cream puffs/Éclair; Crème de menthe; Dessert toppings; Frostings; Fruit leather/rolls; Halvah (candy); Ice cream (vanilla); Ice cream cones; Jams & Preserves; Jellies; Marshmallows; Pies; Pie crust; Popcorn (oil popped); Potato sticks; Puff pastry; Taro chips; Tortilla chips; Potato chips; Frozen yogurt; Honey; Molasses; Popcorn (air popped); Pudding; Chocolate (sweet); Cake (angel food); Peanut butter; Chocolate (dark); Piña colada; Milk shakes; Pancakes; Eggnog; Hot chocolate; Applesauce; Soft (carbonated) drinks; Ginger ale; Tonic water; Pretzels; 80+ proof distilled alc. bev.; Fruit punch; Lemonade; Whiskey; Sports drinks; Malted drinks (nonalcoholic); Coffee; Wine (red); Wine (white); Tea (plain);

Instead <u>choose</u>: Coffee (decaf); Red Bull (drink); Tea (herbal); Water; Beer;

Herbs & Spices, Fast Foods, Prepared Foods

Hot dog; **Syrup (chocolate)**; Breaded shrimp; Cheeseburger; Foie gras or liver pate; French toast; Hash brown potatoes; Hush puppies; Nachos; Onion rings; Pizza; Potato pancakes; Potato salad; Salad dressings; Taco shells; Tahini; Syrup (maple); French fries; Syrup (sorghum); Natto; Hamburger; Syrup (table blends); Egg rolls (veg); Hummus; Sausage (meatless); Teriyaki sauce; Mayonnaise; Cottonseed meal; Tofu (fried); Sugar (brown); Sugar (table, powder); Chicken Nuggets; Soy sauce; Cornmeal (whole-grain); Syrup (malt); Corn cakes; Barbecue sauce; Tofu; Falafel; Sugar (maple); Pickle (sweet); Poppy seed; Cocoa; Sauce (Hoisin); Tempeh; Beef broth & stock; Chicken broth; Soups: beef barley, chicken noodle, veg/beef;

Instead <u>choose</u>: Kimchi; Balsamic vinegar; Herbs & Spices; Capers; Gravies; Horseradish; Mustard; Pickle; Salt; Other Sauces; Sauerkraut; Tomato paste; Vinegar; Succotash; Cole slaw; Ketchup; Macaroni;

Alternative Therapies & Miscellaneous

Excess body weight (obesity in particular can result in VDD); **Cheese made w/whole milk**; Deep-fried foods; Corn syrup; Smoking/Tobacco; 2+ alcoholic drinks/day; Artificial sweeteners; Baking using butter;

Key Nutrients & Herbal Meds

Trans fatty acids; Omega-6 fatty acid (LA); Fat (saturated);

References

All the material and suggestions presented in this book are based on the content available at PersonalRemedies.com. The primary sources used by that web site and therefore this book are US government sources. For complete and detailed information about all the references please visit PersonalRemedies.com.

The suggestions provided are derived from, confirmed by, or based on a long list of references, some of which are listed below. This list does not represent a complete or comprehensive list of all references used. Some references such as the US Government sources are relied upon more than others.

- USDA (US Department of Agriculture). Most of the nutrient data used by Personal Remedies and thus this book are based on USDA publications.
- National Institute of Health (NIH) of the United States. Most of the health information and the relationship between various nutrients and various health conditions are based on NIH and its various publications and agencies.
- NIH - Office of Dietary Supplements Web site.
- MedlinePlus Health Information - a service of National Library of Medicine and NIH.
- NIH - National Institute of Arthritis and Musculoskeletal and Skin Disease
- NIH - National Center for Complementary and Alternative Medicine (NCCAM)
- Dept. of Health and Human Services. Centers for Disease Control and Prevention.
- National Cancer Institute.
- National Diabetes Information Clearinghouse (NDIC). A Service of National Institute of Diabetes and Digestive and Kidney Diseases (NIDDK) and NIH.
- National Kidney and Urologic Diseases Information Clearinghouse (NKUDIC). A service of the National Institute of Diabetes and Digestive and Kidney Diseases (NIDDK), National Institutes of Health (NIH)
- PRAL (Potential Renal Acid Load) formula applied to USDA nutrient database data
- The President's Council on Physical Fitness and Sports.
- US Dept. of Health and Human Services; US Environmental Protection Agency
- Dash Eating Plan; Your Guide to Lowering Blood Pressure with Dash; US Dept. of Health and Human Services; NIH; National Heart, Lung and Blood Institute
- National Heart, Lung and Blood Institute
- Office on Women's Health; US Dept. of Health and Human Services

Secondary sources used by that site include:

- American Heart Association (www.heart.org)
- Institute of Medicine - Food and Nutrition Board - Dietary Reference Intakes. (www.iom.edu)
- *Dietary Reference Intakes - The essential Guide to Nutrient Requirements* (Institute of Medicine of the National Academies. The National Academies Press. 2006)

- *The PDR Family Guide to Natural Medicines & Healing Therapies* (Ballantine Books; New York. First Edition; May 2000)
- *The PDR Family Guide to Nutritional Supplements* (Ballantine Books; New York; 2001)
- MayoClinic.com. Reliable information for a healthier life from Mayo Clinic (www.mayoclinic.com)
- Harvard School of Public Health (www.hsph.harvard.edu)
- American Cancer Society (www.cancer.org)
- American Academy of Physical Medicine and Rehabilitation (www.aapmr.org)
- American Diabetic Association (www.diabetes.org)
- American Dietetic Association (www.eatright.org)
- Multiple Sclerosis Society (www.nationalmssociety.org)
- *The American Pharmaceutical Association Practical Guide to Natural Medicines*. (Andrea Pierce; Morrow; 1999)
- Living Well With HIV/AIDS - A manual on nutritional care and support for people living with HIV/AIDS. Food and Agriculture Organization of the United Nations
- Stanford Hospital & Clinics. Low FODMAP diet handout
- The University of Arizona Campus Health Service. The Low FODMAPs Diet.
- Crohn's & Colitis Foundation of America
- www.herpes.com
- Australian Institute of Sports (www.ais.org.au)
- www.healthandage.com (Sponsored by Boomerang Pharmaceutical Communications)
- www.essense-of-life.com
- Gout (Prof. R. Grahame, Dr. A. Simonds and Dr. E. Carrey); and www.acumedico.com
- Environmental Working Group (www.EWG.org)
- International Foundation for Functional Gastrointestinal Disorders, Inc. (IFFGD), and Monash University, creators of low FODMAP diet for IBS
- Sjögren's Syndrome Foundation (www.sjogrens.org)
- The Dark Side of Wheat (by Sayer Ji; www.GreenMedInfo.com)
- www.GreenMedInfo.com
- High pH therapy research by A.K. Brewer, and Nobel prize winner Otto Warburg (BREWER, A. K. The high pH therapy for cancer tests on mice and humans)
- Linus Pauling Institute Micronutrient Research for Optimum Health
- *Eat Well, Live Well with Spinal Cord Injury* (Joanne Smith and Kylie James; 2013)
- The Oxalate Content of Food By Helen O'Connor, MS, RD
- Oxalate Content of Foods. The Children's Medical Center (Dayton's Children)
- The Oxalosis & Hyperoxaluria Foundation
- New York University (NYU) Langone Medical Center

For Additional Information

For personal food list suggestions for
- other health conditions,
- other combinations of health conditions,
- a greater list of food choices,

and for more detailed nutrition information, you may wish to look at other books in our *Choose This not That* series listed at the end of the book or visit PersonalRemedies.com.

Acknowledgements

We would like to thank the following individuals for their support, encouragement, advice and contributions to the production of this book and contents of the Personal Remedies knowledgebase which is presented in this book: Ester Awnetwant-Esperon, MS, RD, LD; Karen Chiacu-Recco; Kate Fletcher-King; Amanda King; Avirat Kulkarni; Barbara Langathianos; Andrew Lenhardt, MD; Sih Han Lim; Mark Lu, MD; Steve Manson; Art McCray; Dick Neville; Christian Seeber; Nancy Elizabeth Shaw; Diana Silk; Scott Silk; George Sprenkle; Shahin Tabatabaei, MD; Katya Tsaioun, PhD, LD; Foad Vafaei; Rolie Zagnoli; Mory Bahar.

Personal Remedies, LLC

and

Simple Software Publishing

Who is Personal Remedies?

Personal Remedies is the largest producer of health & nutrition apps, books and eBooks for chronic conditions, in the market. Its patented software & knowledgebase can enable organizations such as healthcare providers to deliver apps for personalized and actionable nutrition guidance to their patients suffering from one or multiple chronic conditions.

Who is Simple Software Publishing?

Simple Software Publishing is a small publisher established in 1996. Our passion is to explain complex matters in an easy to understand form. We also strive to minimize the use of paper for production and distribution of books.

Choose This not That Series of Books, eBooks and Apps

Choose This not That for:
- Breast Cancer
- Cancer Prevention
- Cervical Cancer
- Colon Cancer
- Esophageal Cancer
- Gout
- High Blood Pressure
- High Cholesterol
- High Triglycerides
- IBS (Irritable Bowel Syndrome)
- Lung Cancer
- Ovarian Cancer
- Pancreatic Cancer
- Prostate Cancer
- Rheumatoid Arthritis
- Stomach Cancer
- Ulcers
- Vitamin D Deficiency
- … please send us your suggestion!

In addition, we offer mobile apps for the following conditions: age-related macular degeneration (AMD), Alzheimer's disease, celiac disease, Crohn's disease, diabetes type-2, Dietary Guidelines for Americans, Dietary Guidelines for 50+, heart disease, herpes, kidney stones (oxalate), obesity, osteoarthritis, osteoporosis, and PCOS (Polycystic Ovary Syndrome).

How to Order

To order eBooks (on Kindle or Nook) or printed copies of this book, or to order any of our other books please visit Amazon.com, Barnes & Noble, or contact us by email at Publisher@PersonalRemedies.com or send your purchase order or payments to:

Simple Software Publishing
5 Oregon Street
Georgetown, MA 01833

To order a colorful Mobile App version of this book, please visit Apple App store, Google Play (Android), or Amazon App Store.

For suggestions for new books and comments please email us at Books@PersonalRemedies.com.

Progress Tracker

To monitor your progress, date and note your symptoms and relevant data such as triglycerides level in your blood, weight, cholesterol level, blood pressure … below. We love to hear about your feedback and progress. Email us at Books@PersonalRemedies.com.

Made in the USA
Middletown, DE
06 March 2020